AIDS, AFRICA and RACISM

This book demonstrates the racist preconceptions that have guided the collection of evidence on AIDS in Africa and is a timely response to the alleged African origins of AIDS. The authors have added a substantial postscript for this edition. In it they point out that even though several Western researchers have withdrawn some of their evidence and specific claims, they still attempt to substantiate racist hypotheses.

RICHARD CHIRIMUUTA was born in Zimbabwe and became involved in the struggle for independence in his teens. He was deported from Africa in 1972 and has since lived in London. He has written and broadcast widely on African affairs.

ROSALIND CHIRIMUUTA was born in Australia. She came to Britain in 1975 and obtained a diploma in Tropical Medicine and Hygiene, and subsequently specialized in opthalmology. She is a Fellow of the Royal College of Surgeons and now works as a consultant opthalmic surgeon for the National Health Service.

AIDS
AFRICA and RACISM

Richard C. Chirimuuta
Rosalind J. Chirimuuta

'an association in which the free development of each
is the condition of the free development of all'

Free Association Books / London / 1989

Published in 1989 by
Free Association Books
26 Freegrove Road
London N7 9RQ

First published 1987

British Library Cataloguing in Publication Data
Chirimuuta, Richard C.
    AIDS, Africa and racism. – 2nd ed
    1. Africa. Man. AIDS. Reporting by Western
    mass media
    I. Title   II. Chirimuuta, Rosalind J.
    070.4′496169792

ISBN 1-85343-072-2

Printed and bound in Great Britain by
Short Run Press Ltd, Exeter

To our daughter Mazviita and her grandfather,
the late Reverend John Gilbert Harrison,
whom we so sadly miss.

Abbreviations

ARC	AIDS Related Complex
ASFV	African swine fever virus
CDC	Centers for Disease Control
ELISA	Enzyme linked immunosorbent assay
HIV	Human Immunodeficiency Virus
HTLV-I	Human T-Lymphotropic Virus type I
HTLV-II	Human T-Lymphotropic Virus type II
HTLV-III	Human T-Lymphotropic Virus type III
KS	Kaposi's sarcoma
LAV	Lymphadenopathy Associated Virus
MMWR	Morbidity and Mortality Weekly Report
NEJM	New England Journal of Medicine
PCP	Pneumocystis carinii pneumonia
STLV-III	Simian T-cell Lymphotropic Virus III
WHO	World Health Organisation
WER	Weekly Epidemiological Record of the WHO

Contents

Acknowledgements

This book would not have been possible without the assistance and encouragement of many people. We wish to give special thanks to Zimbabwean scientist Davis Gazi, whose penetrating analysis of the AIDS issue provided the inspiration for this book; Dorothy Kuya, Director of Affirmata, whose active and enthusiastic support and advice were crucial to the completion and publication of this work; and Nnamdi Agili, who was always available when needed. A number of African scientists and physicians provided us with reference material and information about the AIDS situation in Africa, and we would particularly like to thank Dr Justinian Ngaiza of the London School of Hygiene and Tropical Medicine. Several African diplomats also gave us moral and practical support. We also wish to thank Stella Russell and Lesley Welch for their comments and advice about the text and Jeff Wynch for proofreading.

Since the book was first published a number of people have provided us with additional information and encouragement, and we would particularly like to thank Dr Felix Konotey-Ahulu, Ankie Hoogvelt, Dr Janie Grote, Heimo Claasen, Duncan Campbell and Les Levidow. And finally we would like to thank Free Association Books for publishing the work.

Introduction

When Europeans first went to Africa to capture slaves for transportation to the new world, they faced a contradiction between the moral principles to which they claimed to adhere and the reality of their daily actions. The philosophy of racism developed to resolve these contradictions, and it is a philosophy which has served the Europeans well throughout the period of slavery and colonialism to the gross economic inequalities between first and third world nations today.

The depth to which racist ideology has penetrated the Western psyche remains profound. The association of black people with dirt, disease, ignorance and an animal-like sexual promiscuity has in no sense been eradicated. When a new and deadly sexually transmitted disease, the Acquired Immune Deficiency Syndrome, emerged in the United States this decade, it was almost inevitable that black people would be associated with its origin and transmission. In this book we contend that the motivation for most of the research into AIDS in Africa has been racist and not scientific. Racism is an irrational system of beliefs without any scientific foundation, and much of the confused, contradictory and simply nonsensical conclusions reached by the scientists about AIDS in Africa can be attributed to their attempts to square their research findings with their racist preconceptions, rather than objective scientific reality.

The homosexual community, under attack from the right wing 'moral majority', quite rightly obtained support from liberal and left wing circles. When black people were attributed with the source of the disease, firstly in Haiti and then central Africa, only their own voices were raised in protest. Fascist organisations, never slow to seize a racist opportunity, went on the propaganda offensive,

1

supported by such unlikely allies as the liberal British newspaper, *The Guardian*, and even the British Communist Party's theoretical journal, *Marxism Today*. Although African journalists and scientists were frequently critical of AIDS research in Africa, these views were completely ignored by the Western media.

In this book we undertake a careful examination of the scientific literature on AIDS in Haiti and Africa. We discuss the difficulties in reaching a clinical diagnosis of AIDS in tropical countries which have a high rate of parasitic and other infectious diseases, and question the reliability of the seroepidemiological studies which have formed the basis of the exaggerated claims of the extent of the AIDS problem in Africa. We examine the way this research has been presented by the mass media both in the West and in Africa. We endeavour to expose the fundamentally flawed nature of the evidence and arguments offered in support of the African hypothesis, and attempt to explode the myth that Africa is at the epicentre of the world AIDS pandemic.

At times we have felt like the boy who shouted that the Emperor had no clothes, but we urge all Africans never to feel overwhelmed by the weight of Western scientific opinion, which has so frequently served the master race and not the truth. We hope this book will be useful to all those who have a genuine interest in combatting this peril that threatens us all.

Derbyshire, Britain   Richard C Chirimuuta
                                                    Rosalind J. Chirimuuta

Chapter 1

The Beginnings of the Epidemic

The Western world is now largely convinced that the Acquired Immune Deficiency Syndrome, or AIDS, originated in Africa, and that Africa is responsible for infecting the world. This conviction is the consequence of several years of "scientific" study reported in the medical journals and relayed to the public by the mass media. It now seems almost incredible that the earliest accounts of the disease, in white American homosexuals,[1] made no reference to Africa, Africans or even travel abroad, and that even today the United States accounts for more than seventy percent of the world's AIDS cases.[2] How is it possible that this predominately American disease has been attributed to the African continent?

The first indication that a new disease had emerged in the world appeared in the *Morbidity and Mortality Weekly Report (MMWR)*, a publication of the Centers for Disease Control (CDC) in Atlanta, Georgia which collects statistics on the incidence of diseases throughout the United States. They reported the occurrence of a rare form of pneumonia, *Pneumocystis carinii*, in five homosexual men in three different hospitals in Los Angeles. The report was followed by this editorial note:

> *Pneumocystis* pneumonia in the United States is almost exclusively limited to severely immunosuppressed patients. The occurrence of pneumocytosis in these 5 previously healthy individuals without a clinically apparent underlying immunodeficiency is unusual. The fact that these patients were all homosexuals suggests an association between some aspect of homosexual lifestyle or disease acquired through sexual contact and *Pneumocystis* pneumonia in this population.[3]

3

By August 1981 it was obvious that something highly unusual was occurring. The CDC documented a total of 108 cases of *Pneumocystis carinii* pneumonia (PCP) and/or Kaposi's Sarcoma (KS), a rare form of cancer, from 1976. The group was described in the following way:

> The majority of the reported cases of KS and/or PCP have occurred in white men. Patients ranged in age from 15-52 years; over 95% were men 25-49 years of age. Ninety-four percent (95/101) of the men for whom sexual preference was known were homosexual or bisexual. Forty percent of the reported cases were fatal. Of the 82 cases for which the month of diagnosis is known, 75 (91%) have occurred since January through July 1981. Although physicians from several states have reported cases of KS and PCP among previously healthy homosexual men, the majority of cases have been reported from New York and California.[4]

This new syndrome came to be known as the Acquired Immune Deficiency Syndrome in the scientific journals and the "Gay Plague"* in the popular press. It was apparent that a major epidemic was underway.

Initial speculations by the doctors as to the cause of the syndrome concentrated on the sexual habits of homosexuals. A high rate of promiscuity, it was thought, could damage the body's immune system. Amyl nitrates, used as sexual stimulants by homosexuals, were at one stage thought to be the cause.[5] As news of this deadly epidemic reached the public, anti-homosexual hysteria, kept at bay by the Gay Rights movement of the previous decade, underwent a new and venomous resurgence. The religious fundamentalists saw AIDS as God's wrath visited on the Sodom and Gomorrah of the homosexual communities of San Francisco, Los Angeles and Manhattan. In his book "AIDS and the New Puritanism", Dennis Altman, a homosexual academic, described the anti-homosexual hysteria and the response of the homosexual community. He provided the following quote from Ronald Godwin of the Moral Majority:

> What I see is a commitment to spend our tax dollars on research to allow these diseased homosexuals to go back to their perverted practices without any standards of accountability.[6]

Even the editor of the US Southern Medical Journal joined in the attack:

> Might we be witnessing, in fact, in the form of a modern communicable disorder, a fulfillment of St. Paul's pronouncement: 'the due penalty for their error'?[7]

Altman cogently perceived the dangers of such bigotry:

Once questions of blame and responsibility for the disease intruded into public discussion, it was clear that AIDS would be political in a way that is unprecedented for a disease in modern times. The vehemence with which homosexuals were attacked for the disease... obscured the reality that this was a new and very dangerous epidemic disease for which no one could be held responsible in any real sense... Neither blame nor guilt is a useful response to an epidemic.[8]

Confronted with a disease that was killing friends and lovers, American homosexuals organised a vigorous response:

The rapidity of the gay response was possible because of a decade of organisation-building among American homosexuals, involving national political groups, such as the National Gay Task Force and the National Gay Rights Advocates, local political groups like the Alice B. Toklas and Harvey Milk Gay Democratic and Log Cabin Republican Clubs in Washington, as well as literally thousands of communal groups offering social, religious, cultural, sporting and business activities. Almost all major American cities now possess extensive gay organizations catering to most conceivable interests, and this is increasingly true for other Western countries.[9]

Trusts were formed to offer advice and support to homosexual AIDS sufferers, to promote sexual practices that would reduce the risk of infection, and to pressure governments to release more funds for research. As Altman states, many of the AIDS researchers themselves were homosexual:

In discussing the response of the medical profession to AIDS it is important to recognize that many of those involved in AIDS research and care are themselves gay.[10]

He recognized that this could cause problems of scientific objectivity:

The fact that so many AIDS researchers are themselves gay — though not often openly so — makes it particularly difficult to maintain scientific "objectivity". (Both prejudice and the desire to avoid prejudice can be involved. Some researchers may well have shied away from certain hypotheses because of a fear of being labelled homophobic).[11]

Although Altman and many other homosexuals quite rightly rejected attempts to blame them for the AIDS epidemic, they uncritically accepted and propagated suggestions that AIDS had originated in black people and was primarily a black and not a homosexual problem:

The most striking indication that AIDS was in no intrinsic sense a disease of homosexuals came in the mounting evidence of its widespread existence in central Africa, where it seemed to have very little correlation with male homosexuality. The connection with Africa was known to researchers as a real possibility from 1982 on, but it took some time to be reported in the mass media, at least in the United States.[12]

Peter Tatchell, another gay activist and left-wing socialist, echoed this view in the British Communist Party weekly, *7 Days:*

> Contrary to the mythology that Aids is a gay plague, the overwhelming majority of people with Aids are heterosexual, including as many women as men and almost as many children as adults. Most of these Aids cases are in central Africa, where the incidence of Aids far surpasses New York or Los Angeles. According to World Health Organisation figures released in June, between five and ten million people have been infected with the virus worldwide. In Africa it is estimated that 6% of the total population is now infected but in some countries it is much higher — 25% of the Malawi population, 23% of the Ugandan population and 18% of the populations of Rwanda and Zambia.[13]

This attempt to deflect anti-homosexual fire onto central Africans shows little respect for either truth or logic. If we consider the figure of 6% of the total African population of 517 million, there would be over 31 million AIDS carriers on the African continent alone, and, estimating from American experience, half a million new cases of AIDS in Africa each year.[14] Our research failed to find a World Health Organisation publication reporting 5 to 10 million carriers in the world, and the WHO world tally of AIDS cases published in November 1986 included only 1,069 African cases.[14] Malawi had not reported a single case of AIDS when Tatchell made his sweeping pronouncements,[15] and even now has seen only 13 cases.[16]

Whilst Altman is prepared to admit "the extent of plain old-fashioned racism, to which gays are no more immune than anyone else"[17], neither he nor any other homosexual organisation or individual has ever raised the possibility of a racist motivation for the Haitian or African hypotheses. Altman discussed the appearance of AIDS in Haitian immigrants "which led researchers to go to Haiti in search of a possible source of the disease"[18] but failed to ask why they should conduct their search in Haiti and not at home. We are told that many of the researchers are homosexual, their scientific objectivity is questionable, and they are no less racist than the rest of white America. Yet Altman accused the Haitians of scapegoating homosexuals when they suggested that AIDS may have been introduced to Haiti by homosexual tourists from the United States, and proffered an extraordinarily offensive alternative explanation:

> One suggestion was that African monkeys, possible carriers of AIDS, were imported into Haiti and kept as pets in male brothels.[19]

Like most western writers on AIDS, Altman's capacity for objectivity or logical thought is overwhelmed by the desire to believe that AIDS originated in black people. This is clearly illustrated by his objections to the removal of Haitians from the official "at risk" list:

> Under pressure, officials began to remove Haitians from the "risk group" classification. In August 1983 the New York City Department of Health ceased to classify Haitians, and in November Haitians were removed from the official "at risk" list of Ontario. In April 1985 the CDC finally dropped Haitians from their list of "groups at high risk", with the comment that "the Haitians were the only risk group that were identified because of who they were rather than what they did.[20]

Even though Altman mentioned that American researchers may have failed to obtain relevant information about homosexuality or drug abuse from their Haitian patients because of language and cultural barriers[21], and quoted research that showed ordinary Haitians were not significantly at risk for AIDS[22], he continued to argue that Haitians were removed from the "at risk" register for political and not scientific reasons:

> What has been distinctive about the classification of Haitians is that, unlike other groups, they protested their classification as a risk group, and even without much clout domestically, their status as a nationality lent a certain support to their claim.[23]

Haitians, it seems, should believe whatever the white folks say in spite of any evidence to the contrary. And particularly when they are being blamed for a deadly new sexually transmitted disease. Racism, like AIDS, is not a very selective disease. It infects liberal academics and fascist scholars alike.

American homosexuals were not the only group looking for a non-American origin for AIDS. Although the "gay plague" theory superficially managed to absolve the rest of America from the stigma of AIDS, the disease was perceived by the rest of the world as an essentially American phenomenon. Soon rumours began to circulate that the AIDS virus had been artificially manufactured in an American laboratory, perhaps for military purposes. Indeed, as Altman stated, the Defense Department discussed the theoretical possibility of such developments as early as 1969:

> Within the next 5 to 10 years it would probably be possible to make a new infective micro-organism which could differ in certain important respects from any known disease-causing organisms. Most important of these is that it might be refractory to the immunological and therapeutic processes upon which we depend to maintain our relative freedom from infectious disease.[24]

Support for a laboratory origin has come from various sources including the Soviet Union, who said the AIDS virus was a biological warfare agent developed by the Central Intelligence Agency and the Pentagon. These charges were rebutted by the American ambassador to Moscow, Arthur Hartman, who wrote to the Soviet magazine *Literaturnaya Gazeta*. His letter was summarised by the US Information Agency:

> The ambassador pointed out that even Soviet scientists agree that AIDS originated in Central Africa and may have existed for several hundred or even several thousand years... (the Soviet articles) are nothing more than a blatant and repugnant attempt to sow hatred and fear among the Soviet population and to abuse a medical tragedy affecting people all over the world, including in the Soviet Union, for base propaganda purposes.[25]

From the standpoint of the AIDS sufferer, blame and guilt may not be useful responses to the epidemic, but when an American ambassador wishes to dissociate his country from the problem, the African connection becomes very useful indeed.

Not every American sought to deny the central role of the United States in the AIDS epidemic. June Osborn, Dean of the School of Public Health at Michigan University, wrote a perceptive article in the New England Journal of Medicine titled "The AIDS Epidemic: Multidisciplinary Trouble". Although she believed in a probable African origin for the virus, Americans, she argued, had spread the virus throughout the world:

> We in the United States have a world-class epidemic on our hands, which we have exported so effectively that the rest of the world is only a little bit behind us... There is a politically interesting aspect of the epidemic that has thus far been mercifully obscure. Although the virus causing AIDS is surely American by adoption, not by birth (the most likely location of transfer to the human species is in Central Africa)**, the epidemic is indeed all-American in its initial dissemination. Most of the rest of the world is catching up with us, with a lag time of two or three years, but the exportations from the United States are easily tracked. We are indeed one world in operational — if not in peaceful — terms. A recent paper from Japan, for instance, documented the absence of antibody from a number of Japanese groups, including homosexuals, but reported 27 percent seropositivity among patients with haemophilia, which was directly related to the American source of the factor VIII and IX concentrates used to treat them. The introduction of AIDS into Denmark and Australia was readily traceable to the return of homosexual men from vacations in New York and San Francisco.[26]

Incredibly the US Government now plans to test potential immigrants for AIDS antibodies, a policy strongly opposed by Dr Osborn and many AIDS researchers.[27] Perhaps the only rational purpose of such tests would be to advise antibody negative would-be immigrants, in the interests of their health, to stay at home!

Fear, ignorance and prejudice and not humanity and rationality have unfortunately characterised our responses to the AIDS epidemic. Although homophobia was the mainstay of the early response to AIDS, to the Western mind black people are the usual repository for fantasies about disease, dirt and sexual promiscuity. It was almost inevitable that, once AIDS appeared in black people in any numbers, they would be attributed with its source. Haiti was the first unfortunate victim. Africa was soon to follow. Let us take a closer look at the scientific evidence for these hypotheses.

Footnotes
*Gay is a term frequently used in the western world for homosexual.
**Using now discredited seroepidemiological data from WC Saxinger et al *"Evidence for Exposure to HTLV-III in Uganda Before 1973"*, Science Vol 227, March 1, 1985, P 1036-8.

References
1. MS Gottlieb, HM Shanker, PT Fan, A Saxon, JD Weisman, I Polanski. *Pneumocystis Pneumonia — Los Angeles.* Morbidity and Mortality Weekly Report, Vol. 30, No. 21, June 5, 1981, p 250-1.
2. *Acquired Immunodeficiency Syndrome (AIDS), Global Data.* WHO Weekly Epidemiological Record No 15, April 10, 1987, p103.
3. op cit MS Gottlieb, HM Shanker et al
4. SM Freidman, YM Felman, R Rothenberg, S Dritz, E Braff, S Fannin, I Heindl, RK Sikes, RA Gunn, MA Roberts. *Follow-up on Kaposi's Sarcoma and Pneumocystis Pneumonia.* Morbidity and Mortality Weekly Report Vol 30, No 33, August 28, 1981, p 409-10.
5. HW Jaffe et al.
    National Case-Control Study of Kaposi's Sarcoma and Pneumocystis carinii Pneumonia in Homosexual Men: Part 1, Epidemiologic Results. Annals of Internal Medicine, August 1983, Vol 99, p145-151.
6. D Altman. *AIDS and the New Puritanism.* Pluto Press, London and Sydney, 1986, p25.
7. ibid p13
8. ibid p25
9. ibid p83
10. ibid p46
11. ibid p41-2
12. ibid p38
13. *7 Days*, October 18,1986.

14. JW Curran, WM Morgan, AM Hardy, HW Jaffe, WW Darrow, WR Dowdle. *The Epidemiology of AIDS: Current Status and Future Prospects.* Science, Vol 229, September 27, 1985 p1352-7.
15. *WHO Weekly Epidemiological Report No 47,* November 21, 1986.
16. *WHO Weekly Epidemiological Report No 3,* January 6, 1987.
17. Altman op cit p100
18. ibid p 37
19. ibid p 72
20. ibid p 72-3
21. ibid p 71
22. ibid p 73
23. ibid p 73
24. ibid p 44
25. Quoted from *The African Guardian*, December 25, 1986, p 15.
26. JE Osborn. *The AIDS Epidemic. Multidisciplinary Trouble.* New England Journal of Medicine, Vol 314 No 12, 1986 p779-82.
27. *The Guardian*, London, June 1, 1987.

Chapter 2

Haiti

Interest in Haiti as the possible source of the American AIDS epidemic was sparked off by a report on AIDS amongst Haitians which appeared in the *Morbidity and Mortality Weekly Report* in 1982. Of the 700 reported cases of AIDS in the United States at that time, 34 were Haitian immigrants, i.e. about 5%.[1] A more detailed account of ten of these Haitians, all of whom were resident in the United States, appeared in the *New England Journal of Medicine* (NEJM) 20th January 1983.[2] At this stage the virus responsible for AIDS had not been identified, nor were specific serological tests available. The authors claimed that all the patients met the criteria for AIDS as defined by the Centers for Disease Control — i.e.:

> A disease, at least moderately predictive of a defect in cell-mediated immunity, occurring in a person with no known cause for diminished resistance to that disease.[3]

The authors summarised their findings as follows:

> We describe acquired immune deficiency manifested by opportunistic infections in 10 previously healthy heterosexual Haitian men. The opportunistic pathogens included *Toxoplasma gondii* (in four patients), *Cryptococcus neoformans* (in one), *Pneumocystis carinii* (in four patients) and *Candida albicans* (in three). Six of the patients also had *Mycobacterium tuberculosis*. Immunologic studies of three patients showed a decrease in the numbers and activity of helper T cells, with normal or increased populations of suppressor T cells. Serologic markers for previous infections from hepatitis A, cytomegalovirus, and herpes simplex virus were detected in several patients. Six of the patients died despite specific antimicrobial therapy. The clinical and immunologic findings in these 10 Haitians are similar to those reported in drug addicts and homosexuals with the acquired immune-deficiency syndrome.[4]

The last sentence is rather interesting. The clinical features of AIDS in the United States were outlined by the Centers for Disease Control in another paper published in the NEJM:

> Of the 2008 cases of AIDS in the United States that were reported to the CDC between June 1981 and August 8, 1983, the most common "marker" diseases have been *P. carinii* pneumonia (1016), Kaposi's sarcoma (533), or both (148). Many other serious opportunistic infections and neoplasms (such as cerebral lymphoma and diffuse, undifferentiated non-Hodgkin's lymphoma) have also been reported. The typical patient with AIDS has multiple opportunistic infections.[5]

Tuberculosis, which is endemic in Haiti, is not a usual clinical feature of AIDS in the United States, yet 6 of the Haitians had this disease. It is a lethal disease in its own right, capable of killing the patient without the assistance of an underlying immune suppression. Toxoplasmosis is also common in Haiti, where it affects up to 33% of the population.[6] Whilst four of the Haitian patients had *P. carinii* pneumonia, only one had multiple opportunistic infections and none had Kaposi's sarcoma. The authors claim that the Haitian cases are clinically similar to the American AIDS cases is not substantiated.

With these dubious clinical criteria, one would expect the diagnosis of AIDS to be supported by substantial laboratory investigations for immune deficiency. This was undertaken in only three patients, and the authors themselves express doubts about the significance of the findings. Antibiotics, including anti-tuberculous drugs, can induce immune suppression:

> However, 5 of the 10 patients received rifampicin for the treatment of tuberculosis for weeks to months before the onset of opportunistic superinfection. Rifampicin is another agent that has been shown to have immunosuppressive effects in vitro and vivo.[7]

Immune supression is a well recognized association of infectious diseases, particularly tuberculosis[8], although the authors are keen to dismiss this possibility:

> However, depressed OKT4/OKT8 ratios are not specific for AIDS, and many diseases, particularly viral infections, can induce an abnormal ratio. It is possible, but highly improbable, that tuberculosis or the therapy for tuberculosis (isoniazid or rifampicin) induced the altered ratios, given the severity of the OKT4/OKT8 abnormality, its similarity to the OKT4/OKT8 abnormalities seen in other AIDS patients, the other accompanying immunologic alterations not usually seen with localised tuberculosis but commonly seen with AIDS, and the presence of other AIDS-associated opportunistic infections...[9]

This is really quite a sleight of hand. Immunological abnormalities are commonly associated with disseminated rather than localised tuberculosis, but at least three of these patients had disseminated disease. In any case, the OKT4/OKT8 ratios for seven of the ten patients were not even estimated. The assumption that all, or even a majority of these patients were suffering from AIDS is far from proven.

But this is not simply a piece of shoddy research. The authors' intentions were clear from the beginning. They were at pains to point out that AIDS was not confined to recognized risk groups:

> This outbreak was unique in that it occurred within a single ethnic group of previously healthy men without histories of homosexuality or drug abuse.[10]

Then, without any scientific evidence, Haitians were accused of infecting America:

> If a viral agent were imported into the U.S. from Haiti by vacationing homosexuals, it might quickly spread within the homosexual community by means of frequent, often anonymous, sexual encounters in bath houses and elsewhere. Homosexual drug addicts, in turn, might introduce the agent via the parenteral route into the heterosexual addict population. To substantiate any hypothesis about the pathogenesis of AIDS with respect to Haitians, we will need to learn more about the Haitian lifestyle in both the U.S. and Haiti. The assumption that heterosexual Haitians and homosexual Americans have little in common may prove erroneous when epidemiologic and anthropologic surveys are completed.[11]

AIDS changed overnight from the "Gay Plague" to the Haitian disease on the basis of such flippant suggestions, which were bound to be disputed. Haitian doctors and researchers replied to this article in the NEJM 9th June, 1983:

> In the Discussion section of the article by Viera et al. concerning the acquired immunodeficiency syndrome (AIDS) in 10 Haitian patients living in the United States, the authors postulated... Haiti as the only possible source of the disease.
>
> Being interested in this problem, we have documented several cases of AIDS in Haiti over the past two years. We share the concern of Viera et al. for the impact on public health of this new disease, which appeared simultaneously in the United States and Haiti. However, we were surprised to see the authors propose such a hypothesis without any scientific basis. Several foci of opportunistic infections have been reported within the homosexual populations in the United States. The hypotheses of a primary source of infection within such groups cannot be excluded. One might readily hypothesize a viral agent introduced into Haiti by vacationing (U.S.) homosexuals and disseminated via a route thus far undefined.[12]

The authors of the original article themselves conceded the points raised in this letter, and cast further doubt on the classification of Haitians as a risk group:

> Although our 10 patients as well as others subsequently described denied homosexuality and drug abuse, one cannot be certain that they had not engaged in these practices and that they were candid when interviewed, because of the stigma associated with homosexuality and drug abuse in the Haitian community.[13]

While these exchanges were taking place in the medical journals, healthy Haitians were being sacked from their jobs and evicted from their homes all over the United States. Haitian criminals were even kept in separate prisons. Being a Haitian literally meant you were treated like an AIDS carrier. "It's more insidious than a person who has been fired or a Haitian who is brought into an emergency room and people get into their space suits," said one Haitian in Miami. "In the minds of a lot of people, Haitians and AIDS go together."[14]

Whilst the American public was indulging in mass anti-Haitian hysteria, scientists were running into difficulties in their attempts to substantiate the Haitian origin. Researchers at the Mount Sinai School of Medicine studied Haitians in New York, comparing them with heterosexual and homosexual Americans:

> Seventeen asymptomatic Haitian-Americans (10 men and 7 women), ranging in age from 26 to 70 years (average 37.3), who have lived in the United States between 1 and 14 years (average 4.2) were studied...
>
> Extensive immunologic studies were done, and the results compared with those obtained in concurrent investigations of 100 clinically well homosexual men and 85 healthy heterosexual men. Although extensive immunologic abnormalities were found among the homosexual men (without AIDS, but in many cases with lymphadenopathy), they were not seen in the Haitians.
>
> ...the results of immunologic tests in the Haitians we studied compare favourably in every respect with the results in normal heterosexual controls in New York City and are significantly different from those in homosexual men in New York.[15]

Another study conducted the following year using the specific blood test for AIDS antibodies found similar results:

> Surprisingly, the rate of HTLV-III seropositivity among Haitian immigrants was found to be less than 5 per cent in a survey conducted in New York City. This relatively low seroprevalence rate is in marked contrast to the rates observed among asymptomatic patients with haemophilia and among homosexual men and parenteral drug users in the New York City area. From these data, it does not appear that being of Haitian extraction by itself, in isolation from other risk factors, increases the relative risk of being exposed to HTLV-III.[16]

Ralph S. Greco of the UMDNJ Rutgers Medical School in New Jersey was moved to write a letter to the Lancet entitled "Haiti and the stigma of AIDS". Greco had worked in Haiti and had regularly visited the island. He argued that AIDS could have been introduced to Haiti by American homosexuals:

> The American media, with the help of some of our colleagues, seems intent on establishing a connection between Haitians and acquired immune deficiency syndrome (AIDS), even though none may exist... During the past five years, Haiti, especially Port-au-Prince, has become a very popular holiday resort for Americans who are homosexual. There are also Haitians who are homosexual, and homosexual prostitution is becoming increasingly common.
>
> Haiti is a poor island. A tiny upper class (which) controls all of the island's wealth and political power is committed to the status quo. For the young Haitian male between the ages of 15 and 30 there is no likelihood of escaping the despair that abounds in Port-au-Prince. As elsewhere, those with money can purchase whatever they want. There is prostitution in Haiti, heretofore heterosexual, and there always will be as long as so many have so little. To admit one's homosexuality is difficult enough in America: in a country like Haiti, where animism and Christianity live side by side, homosexuality or homosexual prostitution will remain a deeply hidden secret.
>
> Haitians can and will continue to acquire AIDS and so will Americans — if they are homosexual, addicted to intravenous drugs, or the recipients of blood products. Being Haitian is not itself a risk factor. However, Haitian Americans have already begun to pay the price for the stigma given them by the media. "Boat people" have been housed in makeshift prisons, and Haitians who have migrated legally are housed in a different "prison" in our ghettos. Some have already lost desperately needed jobs and others are beginning to experience the prejudice of their neighbours who see them not only as black and poor and different but, now, also as contaminated by disease of which they are, rightfully, frightened.
>
> Although it is premature to conclude that homosexuality is a complete explanation of the incidence of AIDS in Haitians, this explanation makes a great deal of sense... Certainly the subject needs to be evaluated by scientists whose agenda is far different from that of the media. In the meantime, I hope we will give these kind and gentle people a respite from this undeserved stigma.[17]

The subject was indeed investigated by scientists in Haiti. They found that AIDS appeared in Haiti at the same time as the United States:

> The recognition of Kaposi's sarcoma and opportunistic infections in Haiti is temporally related to the appearance of AIDS in the United States. The earliest possible case of opportunistic infection in Haiti that is known to our group occurred in July 1978, and the first case of fulminant Kaposi's sarcoma was diagnosed in June 1979. The first cases of Kaposi's sarcoma

and opportunistic infections in homosexual men in the United States were documented in early 1978. We do not believe that AIDS was present in Haiti before 1978. This contention is supported by the clinical experience of the practising pathologists and dermatologists in Haiti and by our inability to identify earlier cases through examination of autopsy and biopsy records. It also seems likely that Haitians would have presented to U.S. hospitals sooner if AIDS had been occurring in Haiti before 1978.[18]

They found that the incidence of AIDS was significantly higher in an area known for male and female prostitution:

The prevalence rate of men with opportunistic infections in Carrefour was significantly higher than that of men in Port-au-Prince (P<0.001 by the chi-square test). This is of interest since Carrefour, a suburb of Port-au-Prince, is recognized as the principal center of male and female prostitution in Haiti.[19]

Of the 61 patients studied, only seven admitted bisexuality, although the authors felt this may have been an underestimate:

There is a very strong bias against homosexuality in Haiti, and our data may underestimate this risk factor.[20]

There was a strong link between the bisexual men and America:

Travel and residence histories of the seven bisexual men indicated that they lived either in Carrefour (four men) or the United States (three). Three had had sexual relations with American men in both Haiti and the United States, and two had had sexual relations with Haitian men with opportunistic infections. Ten of 21 heterosexual men who were questioned said that they had either lived or travelled outside Haiti.[21]

In 1985, two years later, the same researchers reported 229 patients with AIDS in Haiti. They compared them with a control group selected from the patient's friends and siblings, and also sought a history of intramuscular injections. Their findings included the following:

Another difference between the epidemiology of AIDS in Haiti and other countries is the frequency of homosexuality or bisexuality, blood transfusions, and intravenous drug abuse as risk factors. We have identified these factors in 43% of Haitian patients seen between July 1983 and December 1984, which is considerably higher than the 18% we reported in our initial series of 61 patients seen between June 1979 and October 1982. This increase undoubtedly reflects our increased experience in obtaining sensitive information and our use of a more standardized approach, rather than any change in the epidemiology of AIDS in Haiti. In the United States, over 96% of non-Haitian patients with AIDS have the accepted risk factors. In contrast, risk factors have been reported in less than 5% of Haitian-American and African patients.

The disparity in the prevalence of homosexuality and bisexuality, blood transfusion, and intravenous drug abuse in the United States, Haiti, and Africa prompted our search for other potential risk factors or alternate means of transmission of the syndrome. It is a common practice in Haiti for persons to obtain intramuscular injections when they are "not feeling well"... (and) may be given by either medical personnel or piqurists (untrained injection givers). Disposable needles and syringes are not readily available in Haiti, so needles and syringes may be reused without sterilization. During the five year period before the onset of AIDS symptoms, intramuscular medications were received by 89% of the patients and by only 66% of their siblings and friends. The patients also received a larger number of injections annually and were more likely to receive them from nonmedical sources.[22]

These observations are interesting. Great emphasis was placed in the American scientific literature on the low incidence of risk factors, particularly homosexuality, amongst Haitian patients. It seems likely that Haitians were not revealing their sexual preferences to the American doctors. The researchers in Haiti offer the following explanation for the transmission of AIDS into the heterosexual population, which, as we will see later, may also apply to Africa:

...almost all the Haitians with AIDS in our study who had sex with other men were bisexual, which would provide a means for increased heterosexual transmission of AIDS in Haiti.[23]

Other risk factors found amongst the AIDS sufferers included an increased incidence of venereal disease and heterosexual promiscuity (again with parallels to the African situation) and the authors conclude:

At present, we have no evidence to suggest that the syndrome is transmitted by any mechanism other than those that have been recognized to date — homosexual and heterosexual activity, blood transfusions, and the use of contaminated needles and syringes...[24]

Whilst doctors in Haiti were studying the medical evidence, Americans anxious to prove that AIDS had originated in Haiti were indulging in flights of fancy. In a letter to *The Lancet* in April 1983, Jane Teas of the Harvard School of Public Health had enquired, "Could the AIDS agent be a new variant of African swine fever virus?" She wrote:

Closely paralleling the onset of the first cases of AIDS in 1978 in Haiti was the first confirmed appearance of the African swine fever virus (ASFV) also in Haiti, in 1979... In 1976, ASFV was confirmed in Cuba and all pigs were killed. The island remained disease-free until 1980, when the virus reappeared, coincident with the arrival of Haitian refugees. ...Perhaps an infected pig was killed and eaten either as uncooked or undercooked meat. One of the people eating the meat who was both immunocompromised and homosexual would be the pivotal point, allowing for the disease to spread amongst the vacationing 'gay' tourists in Haiti.[25]

Note that Dr Teas proposed that a homosexual Haitian passed the virus to a 'gay' U.S. tourist. Gay is a polite term for homosexual. Haitians were homosexual, but Americans were 'gay'. It seems extraordinary that such a ridiculous hypothesis ever saw the light of day in a scientific publication. As a Zimbabwean scientist, Dr D. Gazi, pointed out:

> Indeed about this time some leading medical journals had decided to give preferential reporting to AIDS articles. This carte blanche was received with both hands by competent and mediocre researchers alike.[26]

There were several replies to this article. A group of Belgian and Dutch doctors tested Dr Teas' hypothesis on seven of their AIDS patients. None of these patients had antibodies to the African Swine Fever Virus, and they concluded:

> Our results, however, make it unlikely that ASFV and the AIDS agent will be found to be related.[27]

A letter was sent to *The Lancet* from Roland St John of the Pan American Health Organisation. He wrote:

> ...I take issue with her explanation of a possible cycle for the accidental introduction of ASFV into the human population. She speculates that, through an improbable series of events, AIDS originated in Haiti. There is no epidemiological evidence to support this idea. Allegations, without strong supporting epidemiological evidence, that one country is responsible for introducing an illness are reminiscent of syphilis in the Middle Ages, when the French worried about the "Italian disease", and vice versa... The danger is that unwarranted speculation of this sort will create a defensive atmosphere in the "accused" country. Haitian physicians have been investigating AIDS in Haiti and have established cooperative research programmes with scientists from other countries, and such cooperation is very important in the search for the cause and means of prevention of the disease.[28]

Such criticisms apply equally well to subsequent events in Africa. Dr St John, though, seems only concerned that such idle speculations would hinder research, and makes no mention of the plight of the Haitians. This was left to a group of doctors in Haiti, who had tested Dr Teas' hypothesis and came up with negative results. They concluded:

> The hypothesis that AIDS originated in Haiti has been raised at least twice

without any scientific basis. Such speculation is damaging to Haiti and Haitian communities abroad.[29]

Another letter of complaint was written by no less than the Haitian ambassador to Washington, Fritz N. Cineas. The letter reads:

The Republic of Haiti has suffered a great injustice over the past year in the American press. Countless broadcast and print journalists have related stories attributing the origins of the acquired immunodeficiency syndrome (AIDS) to Haitians, without sufficient factual data to support this theory. Recently, press reports have reflected a shift in opinion about the origins of the disease. Unfortunately the new evidence often has been hidden on the inner pages, while damaging information about the alleged Haiti-AIDS connection has appeared in front-page stories of American newspapers and journals.

...The volume of media stories relating Haitians and AIDS has cast a pall of gloom over the country, deterring potential business investors and tourists from venturing too near. The negative impact on our already distraught economy has been tremendous.

It is puzzling to contemplate the reasons for selecting Haiti as a target for origination of the dreaded AIDS problem. We sympathise with all AIDS sufferers and hope a cure will be found before hundreds more fall prey to this deadly menace. Haiti however has enough problems without being selected as a scapegoat for a mysterious ailment that has sadly descended on the American homosexual community.

We, as a black nation, well understand the pains of world discrimination and trust that a free, democratic system like the U.S. would be particularly careful to ensure that its medical conclusions are based on objective, thoroughly researched conclusions and not on biased conjecture.

The time is well overdue for the record to be set straight regarding AIDS and the Haiti connection. I am sure responsible institutions like yours will uphold your admirable American tradition of unveiling the truth.[30]

With true American subtlety, this letter was followed by a reminder that went something like, "Letters to the editor should be typed, double spaced (including references) with conventional margins, etc."

Support for America's case against Haiti came from countries around the world. The French reported the case of a French geologist who had received a blood transfusion in Haiti in 1978 after a car accident. The man developed symptoms of AIDS 4 years later, and died within a year.[31] Doctors at another Parisian hospital reported the cases of a Haitian couple.[32] The wife was said to have developed AIDS in August 1981, and died in February 1982. The husband was then admitted to hospital in October 1982, suffering from fever and diarrhoea, and died four months later. Although they were living in Paris at the time of their deaths, the wife had lived in New Jersey where she had sexual relations with another Haitian with AIDS. This phenomenon is called clustering, i.e. the disease could be traced to a group of Haitians in France and America. The same hospital, the Claude Bernard, reported the case of a 24 year-old Haitian woman referred from Guadelope, a French colony in the Caribbean.[33] She died a month after admission with Kaposi's sarcoma and multiple infections. The Canadians reported a Haitian woman who died in 1981 of undifferentiated lymphoma and miliary tuberculosis six weeks after the birth of her child.[34] The infant died several months later of multiple infections. Even the South Africans managed to find a Haitian who, they said, returned to Mozambique.[35]

Despite the concerted efforts in America and abroad, the Haitian hypothesis could not be substantiated. Yet the belief that AIDS had originated in black people was too attractive to abandon. Kevin M. de Cock, a clinical fellow of the University of Southern California, published a lengthy article for debate in the British Medical Journal in August 1984. This article is important for two reasons. Firstly, it vigorously refuted the Haitian hypothesis; and secondly, it was widely quoted in what has come to be known as the African connection, which we will discuss in subsequent chapters. On the Haiti issue, he argued that the disease was most probably introduced to Haiti from the United States:

> The present outbreak of Kaposi's sarcoma and opportunistic infections in the United States began in 1978 although isolated cases may have occurred even earlier. AIDS in the United States would seem to antedate that in Haiti... If AIDS were traditionally endemic in Haiti, one would have also expected it to occur in the neighbouring Dominican Republic.. AIDS was probably introduced to Haiti by vacationing American homosexuals for whom the island was a fashionable resort in the late 1970's... Interestingly, Haitian born patients with AIDS are the only group in the U.S. in whom AIDS has become proportionately less prevalent compared with others at high risk."[36]

For those who still clung to the Haiti story the burial of the myth could be said to have taken place on June 27, 1985 when researchers from the Centers for Disease Control, the University of Miami Medical School and Port-au-Prince published their findings on "Prevalence of HTLVIII/LAV antibodies among Haitians":

> Serum samples collected in July 1982 from 68 Haitian patients seen consecutively over three working days at a private general laboratory in Port-au-Prince, Haiti, and from 28 Haitian personnel who worked in the laboratory, were tested for HTLVIII/LAV Antibody at the Centers for Disease Control by an enzyme linked immunosorbent assay (ELISA)... The prevalence of antibodies to HTLVIII/LAV in these two Haitian

groups was as much as 6 to 30 times lower than that reported for groups at risk for AIDS.[37]

Faced with this overwhelming lack of evidence for a Haitian origin, the Centers for Disease Control ceased to classify Haitians as a high risk group. Needless to say, the truth about the Haitian "origin" never made the press headlines. The newspapers and television were busy writing new scripts on the latest theory — the African Connection.

References

1. *Opportunistic infections and Kaposi's Sarcoma among Haitians in the United States.* Morbidity and Mortality Weekly Report, 1982, Vol 31, p353-4 and 360-1.
2. J Viera, E Frank, TJ Spira, SH Landesman. *Acquired Immune Deficiency Syndrome in Haitians.* New England Journal of Medicine Vol 308 No 3, Jan 20, 1983, p125-9.
3. ibid J Viera, E Frank et al
4. ibid J Viera, E Frank et al
5. JW Curran. *AIDS — Two Years Later.* New England Journal of Medicine Vol 309, 1983, p609-11.
6. *Harrison's Principles of Internal Medicine, 6th edition.* McGraw-Hill Book Company, 1970, p1040.
7. op cit J Viera, E Frank et al
8. op cit *Harrison's Principles of Internal Medicine,* p875.
9. op cit J Viera, E Frank et al
10. ibid J Viera, E Frank et al
11. ibid J Viera, E Frank et al
12. M Bouncy, AC Laroche, B Liautuad et al. *Acquired Immunodeficiency in Hatians.* New England Journal of Medicine, June 9, 1983, Vol 308 No 23, p1419-20.
13. J Viera, E Frank, S Landesman. New England Journal of Medicine, 1983, Vol 308 No 23, p1420.
14. D Altman *AIDS and the New Puritanism.* Pluto Press, 1986, p74.
15. P Nicholas, J Masci, J de Catalogne et al. *Immune Competence in Haitians living in New York.* New England Journal of Medicine, Nov 10, 1983, Vol 309 No 19 p1187-8.
16. SH Landesman, HM Ginzburg, SH Weiss. *Special Report The AIDS Epidemic.* New England Journal of Medicine, Feb 21, 1985, Vol 312 No 8, p521-5.
17. RS Greco. *Haiti and the stigma of AIDS.* The Lancet, August 27, 1983, p515-6.
18. JW Pape, B Liautuad. F Thomas, J-R Mathurin et al. *Characteristics of the Acquired Immunodeficiency Syndrome (AIDS) in Haiti.* New England Journal of Medicine, Oct 20, 1983, Vol 309 No 16 p945-9.
19. ibid JW Pape, B Liautuad. F Thomas, J-R Mathurin et al

20. ibid JW Pape, B Liautuad. F Thomas, J-R Mathurin et al

21. ibid JW Pape, B Liautuad. F Thomas, J-R Mathurin et al

22. JW Pape, B Liautuad, F Thomas, J-R Mathurin et al. *The Acquired Immuno Deficiency Syndrome in Haiti.* Annals of Internal Medicine, 1985, Vol 103, p674-78.

23. ibid JW Pape, B Liautuad, F Thomas, J-R Mathurin et al

24. ibid JW Pape, B Liautuad, F Thomas, J-R Mathurin et al

25. J Teas. *Could AIDS agent be a new variant of African swine fever virus?* The Lancet, April 23, 1983, p923.

26. D Gazi. *The Facts and Myths of AIDS.* (pamphlet)

27. J Colaert, J Desmyter, J Goudsmit, N Clumeck, C Terpstra. *African swine fever virus not found in AIDS patients.* The Lancet, May 14, 1983, p1098.

28. RK St John. *AIDS and African swine fever.* The Lancet, July 9, 1983, p110.

29. E Arnoux, JM Guerin, R Malebranche et al. *AIDS and African swine fever.* The Lancet, July 9, 1983, p110.

30. FN Cineas, Ambassador, The Republic of Haiti. *Haitian Ambassador deplores AIDS connection.* New England Journal of Medicine, Sept 15, 1985, Vol 309 No 11 p668-9.

31. T Andreani, Y Le Charpentier, J-C Brouet et al. *Acquired Immunodeficiency with intestinal Cryptosporidiosis: Possible transmission by Haitian whole blood.* The Lancet, May 28, 1983, p1187-91.

32. E Dourin, C Penalba, M Wolfe et al. *AIDS in a Haitian couple in Paris.* The Lancet, May 7, 1983, p1040-1.

33. B Autran, I Gorin, M Leibowitch et al. *AIDS in a Haitian woman with cardiac Kaposi's sarcoma and Whipples disease.* The Lancet, April 2, 1983, p767.

34. JH Joncas, G Delange, Z Chad, N Lapointe. *Acquired (or congenital) immunodeficiency of infants born of Haitian mothers.* New England Journal of Medicine, April 7, 1983, Vol 308 No 14 p842.

35. *The Advisory Group on AIDS Update on AIDS.* South African Medical Journal, November 8, 1986, Vol 70 p639.

36. KM De Cock. *AIDS: An old disease from Africa?* British Medical Journal, August 4, 1984, Vol 289 p306-8.

37. AE Pichenik, TJ Spira, R Elie et al. *Prevalence of HTLV/LAV antibodies among Haitians.* New England Journal of Medicine, Vol 312 No 26 p1705.

Chapter 3

Early African Cases

As the Haitian hypothesis was falling out of favour, reports began to appear in the scientific literature of cases of AIDS in patients who originated from central Africa, or in Europeans who had travelled or lived in central African countries. An interesting feature of these reports is that they never appeared during the Haiti episode although they all seem to predate known Haitian cases.

A paper widely quoted as confirming the presence of AIDS in Africa prior to the American epidemic is "AIDS in a Danish Surgeon (Zaire, 1976)" by I. C. Bygbjerg published in *The Lancet* April 1983. It was, like most reports of AIDS in Africans, sent as a letter to the editor, thus avoiding the normal strict editorial assessment designed to assure scientific validity. In the introductory paragraph the author states:

> Little attention has been paid to the hyperendemic focus of KS (Kaposi's Sarcoma) in central Africa. Cases of AIDS without KS stand little chance of being detected locally because immunological laboratories are not available. Three acutely deadly viruses of central African origin have been discovered in recent years (Lassa, Marburg, and Ebola viruses). Lancet letters from Belgium... and France... on AIDS/Kaposi's sarcoma among former residents of central Africa (Zaire and Chad) may justify the following questions — is there a connection between African and American AIDS/KS; is the underlying cause another deadly, but slow-acting, African virus introduced to America, perhaps via Haiti; and was the patient in the following case the victim of such an agent?[1]

These few sentences contain so many inaccuracies that we are unable to do justice to them all. Quite contrary to the author's assertion, the endemic form of KS is not associated with AIDS,[2,3,4,5] and the appearance of the aggressive form of KS in the early 1980's was

23

recognized by local physicians as a new phenomenon.[6,7] Bygbjerg conjures up an image of central Africa as a hot-house for new, deadly viruses. The *Lassa* virus is a west African virus and is not found in central Africa, but is related to the *Junin* and *Machupo* viruses in Argentina and Bolivia respectively.[8] Deadly viruses have been found throughout the world, for example the *Murray Valley encephalitis* virus in Australia, and the *St Louis encephalitis* virus in the United States.[9] The extraordinary suggestion of a Zaire/Haiti connection has been raised by many researchers, and is entirely a product of their imaginations. Lastly, although the letter is widely quoted as evidence that Zairean AIDS predated the cases in the United States, and as proof of the African origin of AIDS, in the final sentence of the first paragraph even the author has his doubts. How, then, was the letter titled "AIDS in a Danish surgeon". Surely this is mischievous to say the least. But what of the case itself?

The previously healthy Danish woman who worked in Zaire from 1972 to 1977, suffered from chronic diarrhoea during most of her stay in Zaire, but in in 1976 developed fatigue, wasting and generalised lymphadenopathy, *Pneumocystis carinii* pneumonia and other opportunistic infections and died the following year. The authors suggest she may have acquired the infection from her patients:

> She could recall coming across at least one case of KS while working in northern Zaire, and while working as a surgeon under primitive conditions she must have been heavily exposed to blood and excretions of African patients.[10]

This is an interesting proposal. There is no evidence that the AIDS virus was responsible for the endemic form of KS in equatorial Africa, and at the time of this patient's illness and death AIDS had not been described and there was no recognised association between *Pneumocystis carinii* pneumonia and Kaposi's sarcoma. One begins to wonder whether some of the history from the patient was obtained posthumously. Another article titled "AIDS — two years later" published in the *New England Journal of Medicine* the same year commented:

> No cases have been documented among health-care or laboratory workers who have had clear-cut exposure to patients with AIDS and no other risk factors. The future occurrence of such cases remains a theoretical possibility, but the lack of related cases more than four years after the first AIDS cases were seen suggests that the risk is minimal.[11]

Three such cases have since been reported, and none has died.[12,13] Another disease that is very common in rural Zaire, hepatitis B, is readily transmitted by contact with patient's blood but the Danish surgeon was apparently unaffected. Tests on blood collected in Zaire prior to the early 1980's have failed to demonstrate the presence of AIDS antibodies.[14,15] Transmission of the AIDS virus from patient to doctor seems highly improbable.

Dr Bygbjerg concluded his letter in the anecdotal manner typical of many western researchers involved with Africa:

> During my stay in Zaire in 1976 I was impressed by the epidemiological and virological flying teams from the USA and Europe who quickly identified Ebola virus. Perhaps such teams should search for another African virus, albeit slow killing, and explore the possible connection between endemic and epidemic AIDS/KS in Africa and America. Because of the frequency in the US homosexual community of infections usually seen only in the tropics, Manhattan got the name 'tropical isle' as early as 1968. This name is appropriate today and may even point to the origin of AIDS/KS.[16]

As we said before, KS is not AIDS, and there is no connection between Zaire and Manhattan except in the mind of the author. Such unscientific writing would be inappropriate for the columns of a medical correspondent of a newspaper, let alone a scientific publication.

Incidently, the preceding letter in the same journal was an account of a West German homosexual who developed an AIDS-like illness in 1976. Unlike "AIDS in a Danish surgeon" it is accurately titled "Kaposi's sarcoma, aplastic pancytopaenia, and multiple infections in a homosexual (Cologne, 1976)" This patient had not visited the United States, Haiti or Africa. The authors conclude:

> This patient's Kaposi's sarcoma and homosexuality may have been fortuitous and unrelated to the current epidemic of AIDS — or his Kaposi's sarcoma may have been a consequence of AIDS, a hypothesis supported by the non-bacterial meningitis and perianal condylomata.[17]

Although both patients developed their illnesses in the same year the Danish article is widely quoted and the German largely ignored. Yet Zaireans and not Germans are accused of infecting the world.

The following is an extract from a letter co-authored by three Belgian doctors:

> Three independent groups in Paris and Brussels have recently reported on severe opportunistic infections in previously healthy Africans, immigrants or not, without history of drug abuse, transfusions, or homosexuality. In all three reports these were patients from Zaire and it was suggested that Central Africa may be an endemic area for the supposed infectious agent(s) of AIDS. Over the past two years at least a dozen Zairean patients have been admitted to hospitals in Belgium with clinical features suggestive of AIDS...Since only the better off families

of Zaire can afford medical care in Europe these patients may just be the tip of the epidemiological iceberg. For about two years (i.e. since 1981) there has been a sharp increase in cryptococcosis in the major hospitals of Kinshasa...[18]

The authors are suggesting that the AIDS epidemic began in Zaire in 1981, however their aims seem to be in another direction:

We describe here probable AIDS in a Zairean seen here (i.e. Belgium) four years before the syndrome was first described in the USA.[19]

Like the case of the Danish doctor, "probable" AIDS becomes a definite case of AIDS in 1977 in the title of the letter, and is subsequently quoted elsewhere in support of a Zairean origin for the virus. The assertion that this case predates American cases by four years is simply not true, as retrospective American cases have been reported from 1978.[20] This information was readily available, but these eminent doctors preferred to remain wilfully ignorant of such cumbersome facts. The patient died of disseminated *Cryptococcis neoformans*, and the authors themselves state that the immunological evaluation was incomplete. The patient's child was also found to have a depressed cell-mediated immune response, but the immune status was normal when retested two years later. If it was indeed AIDS that killed the mother, is the child the first human to recover from the disease?

With sightings of African cases in France and Belgium, other former colonial powers in Africa were not to be denied. A group of three London hospitals reported that they had seen a Ugandan AIDS case.[21] Although this woman had lived in the United Kingdom since 1963, the authors were at pains to point out that she had visited Uganda in 1979 where they presumed she had contracted the disease. According to the authors the patient fulfilled the clinical criteria for a diagnosis of AIDS, yet they state there was no history of promiscuity, drug abuse or blood transfusion and offer no alternative explanation as to how she became infected. Is a visit to Uganda a sufficient explanation? Although the authors say she was married with three children, no mention is made of the immune status of her husband and children. If the patient was reticent about her private life, why could she not have caught the disease in the United Kingdom.

Another British case was titled "HTLV-III infection and AIDS in a Zambian nurse resident in Britain."[22] This nurse had been resident in Britain for three years when she developed clinical features of AIDS and died of fulminating cerebral toxoplasmosis. She is reported to have had no recent sexual contact, although the authors do not say whether she had been celibate in Britain, nor is any other account given of her sexual history in Zambia. By implication simply coming from Zambia is reason to acquire the disease, yet seroepidemiological studies have shown that the virus was rare in Zambia in the early 1980's.[23] Although this patient was seropositive for HIV, the tests used are not mentioned, and Africans are known to give a high rate of false positivity to some of the tests.

Another group of British doctors reported the case of a 49 year-old white Englishwoman who they believe caught AIDS from her African ex-husband:

> The patient had been married to a Ghanaian businessman for 18 years, but had been divorced from him for four years before admission, last sexual intercourse having taken place between them in December 1979. Anal intercourse had not taken place at any time. She had never had any other sexual contacts and had no history of intravenous drug abuse or blood transfusion. She had lived in Ghana between 1963 and 1965, but apart from a visit to Lusaka, Zambia, in 1978 had not returned to Africa since. Her ex-husband had lived only in Ghana, Britain, and latterly Zambia (from 1975). In 1978 he returned from Lusaka, after which his wife developed gonorrhoea... The most likely explanation for the development of AIDS in this patient is that she was infected with HTLV-III through sexual intercourse with her ex-husband by 1979. It must be assumed that the husband is an asymptomatic carrier and himself contracted HTLV-III infection in Zambia, where there is evidence of an AIDS like epidemic.[24]

Why must we make such assumptions? In support of their argument, the authors state:

> Further, it has been suggested that the agent causing AIDS, currently believed to be HTLV-III, may exist in a stable equilibrium in an African environment but alters its expression in a new population.[25]

Presumably they are attempting to explain why the husband has remained healthy, but surely there is a contradiction between a "stable equilibrium in an African environment" and an "AIDS-like epidemic" in Zambia. In fact the Zambian epidemic is well documented and began in 1983, five years after the husband left the country. Without interviewing the husband, the authors are in no position to assume that he was a carrier, and if so, where he may have contracted AIDS (perhaps London, or during a stopover in Frankfurt or Rome), or even that he was exclusively heterosexual. Yet logical thought is never the hallmark of scientists trying to prove the African connection. The authors' intentions are clear in the final paragraph:

> This case illustrates the need for clinicians to consider the diagnosis of AIDS in all patients, even if they do not obviously fall into the most

common risk groups. We believe it supports the hypothesis that AIDS may have its origins in central Africa. Furthermore, it indicates the need for a full travel history in both patient and sexual partners as well as a full sexual history in the evaluation of patients who might have AIDS.[26]

One of the authors of this paper is Dr A J Pinching, senior lecturer in clinical immunology at St Mary's Hospital Medical School. He has always been a leading proponent of the African connection, irrespective of the contradictions between the different arguments on offer. For example in this paper, black people are apparently resistant to AIDS but are infecting white people with whom they have sexual contact. Yet he has recently published research (May 1987) "proving" that central Africans, from unspecified countries, have a genetic predisposition for developing AIDS.[27] For scientists like Dr Pinching, where there is a will there will always be a way.

"AIDS in a black Malian" (who had been a French resident since 1973) was reported by the Claude Bernard Hospital in Paris. The patient was a 35 year old man who fell ill in 1981. He visited his homeland after this initial illness (between May and September 1982). The authors observe that:

> ...AIDS in a black Malian who had never been to central Africa suggests that the epidemiological frontiers of the AIDS agent are not yet closed.[28]

How AIDS in a Malian resident in France for many years implicates Mali is perhaps best known to the authors.

From the beginning of the AIDS epidemic, the French have been amongst the most vociferous supporters of a black connection, first Haiti and then central Africa. In support of this alleged connection, the Bureau of Epidemiology in Paris in 1983 published details of the their first 29 confirmed cases of AIDS:

> The first French case of unusual opportunistic infection was observed in a young male homosexual in July, 1981, and further cases of the acquired immunodeficiency syndrome (AIDS) led to the creation of a multidisciplinary group of physicians whose first purpose was to evaluate this syndrome in France... Between March 31 and Dec 29, 1982, 29 confirmed cases were reported to the study group... All patients except 2 came from the Paris area... three geographical locations were often implicated (the USA, Haiti, and equatorial Africa)... More striking (than Haiti) is the association with equatorial Africa... We suggest that Equatorial Africa is an endemic zone for the supposed infectious agent(s) of this illness.[29]

So what is the evidence for an African connection? As with so many articles on AIDS in Africa, an inspection of the data provided simply does not confirm the claims. Ten patients had visited Africa: a Zairean couple, 7 French citizens and one Portuguese man. The countries visited were listed as follows: 3 Maghreb, 1 Egypt and Ivory

Coast, 1 Mozambique and Angola, 3 Zaire, 1 Morocco. This is really quite odd. The countries of the Maghreb are Tunisia, Algeria and Morroco (although the authors list Morocco separately) and they are certainly not in equatorial Africa. Neither is Egypt, Mozambique or much of Angola, nor had any of these countries reported cases of AIDS in 1983. So we are left with only three people with an equatorial African connection. Six of the ten patients were homosexuals, and all but one had visited countries other than Africa, so there are only 4 patients (2 Zaireans, a Portuguese man and a French woman) who had visited Africa and had no other risk factors, and we do not know if the Portuguese man and French woman had actually been to equatorial Africa. From this shoddy piece of statistical analysis the French concluded that central Africa was an AIDS endemic area.

The majority of the early African AIDS cases in Europe were Zaireans reported from Belgium.[30] Five of these cases were reviewed in *The Lancet*, March 1983,[31] and an expanded version of the report appeared in the *New England Journal of Medicine* in 1984 co-authored by no less than 14 Belgian doctors:

> In a preliminary report we suggested that black Africans from Equatorial Africa might be another high risk group. In this paper we extend our observations and describe demographic, clinical, immunologic, and serologic characteristics of 22 black Africans and one white man who had been living in Zaire. Eighteen had opportunistic infections or Kaposi's sarcoma, and five had symptoms consistent with the prodromal phase of AIDS.[32]

The report is full of conflicting ideas. Not surprisingly the authors emphasise the Zairean rather than the Belgian connection of these patients:

> All patients were of upper socioeconomic status. Eight had been living in Zaire and came to Belgium because of unexplained weight loss and chronic diarrhoea. The other 10 had been living in Belgium for 4 to 48 months (median 17) at diagnosis but had frequently returned to Africa for familial or business purposes.[33]

Of the 23 cases reviewed only one was diagnosed (retrospectively) in 1979, and the remaining cases were diagnosed in 1981 and 1983. This is well into the American AIDS epidemic. The diagnosis of AIDS in a number of these patients seems rather tenuous. Three patients had evidence of tuberculosis, and nine had parasitic infections, including ankylostomiasis, schistosomiasis, amebiasis, ascaridiasis and filariasis. Three patients had cerebral toxoplasmosis, and five other patients had evidence of current or previous *Toxoplasma gondii* infection. The authors recognize that parasitic diseases can induce immune suppression, but dismiss this possibility in their patients:

> Parasitic disease and malnutrition are two possible causes of immunodepression in Africa. A wide range of prevalent protozoal and helminthic infestations have been reported to induce immunodeficiency. In malaria the number of lymphocytes is reduced but cell mediated immunity seems to be unaffected and only humoral immunity is impaired. African trypanosomiasis has been shown to be associated with several T-cell dysfunctions. Diffuse cutaneous leishmaniasis is known to induce immunosuppression, but it is restricted to parasite-specific antigens. On the basis of repeated examinations of blood and stool specimens, as well as serologic tests, we were able to exclude active parasitic infestations as a possible cause of the impaired cell-mediated immunity in all our subjects except patient 11...[34]

The authors fail to mention that other infectious diseases, including tuberculosis[35] and cytomegalovirus infection[36], can also induce immune suppression. Amongst the 18 cases of "AIDS" we find a patient with cytomegalovirus infection only, another with cerebral toxoplasmosis only, a third with tuberculosis and toxoplasmosis (neither of which are strictly opportunistic infections), and a patient with idiopathic pneumonia and *Candida albicans* stomatitis which the authors themselves describe as "probable AIDS". It would seem that simply being a central African increases the risk of being classified as an AIDS patient, irrespective of the patient's true state of health.

The authors are unable to dismiss the possibility that malnutrition was responsible for immune suppression in their patients:

> Our patients were previously healthy adults in the upper socio-economic class. Thus it is unlikely that malnutrition was the primary cause of their syndrome. However since most of them presented with severe loss of weight it is possible that malnutrition was an aggravating factor.[37]

Towards the end of the article, we find another example of confused European thinking that can only envisage viral transmission from black to white people:

> The occurrence of AIDS in black Africans who lived in Belgium or Central Africa and who had not been exposed to other risk factors for the disease may signify that the putative agent of AIDS is endemic both in Europe and Africa. However, a European reservoir is unlikely. Indeed, until now, all reported European cases occurred in high-risk subjects (homosexual men, patients with haemophilia, and those who had had blood transfusions) who had travelled to the United States or the Caribbean region or had received blood products from these countries. All our African patients living in Belgium traveled regularly to their country of origin and may have acquired the syndrome there, since it occurred in those who later came to Belgium for medical care.[38]

The assumption here is that there are no significant links between Zaire and the United States, when in fact Zaire has closer ties with the U.S. than virtually any other African country, for example housing the headquarters for the American Central Intelligence Agency's covert actions for the whole of sub-Saharan Africa.[39,40] The authors are also assuming that Belgians, once infected, are incapable of infecting Zaireans, and that infected Zaireans will not spread the disease once they return home. Yet whilst the Belgians would like to believe that AIDS is an old African disease, they feel obliged to express some doubts:

> Concerning cryptococcosis, from 1953 to 1967, only 14 cases were reported from Zaire, whereas in 1981 and 1982 15 cases of fatal cryptococcal meningitis occurring in young Zaireans were diagnosed in the Mama Yemo Hospital of Kinshasa.
>
> It is possible that AIDS has always been present but unrecognised in Africa. However we are struck by the increasing number of patients who have come from Zaire or Rwanda to Belgium during the past four years to seek medical care. We believe that AIDS is a new disease that is spreading in central Africa.[41]

Even the Swedes, with no African colonial ties, were not to be denied. They wrote to *The Lancet:*

> We want to add some important data to a case-report in The Lancet and elsewhere. The patient was a white Scottish heterosexual male who had been working in Kenya and Tanzania for 3 years and who died of acquired immunodeficiency syndrome (AIDS) in Glasgow in December, 1982. The absence of risk factors for AIDS, including a history of exposure to blood or blood products, was emphasised. In the light of our experience with this patient, the Glasgow workers' assumption that simply "working in" East Africa is associated with an increased risk for AIDS needs further comment.
>
> 1 year before his admission to hospital in Glasgow he was admitted to Roslagstull Hospital, Stockholm, with lymphadenopathy, splenomegaly and wasting. No diagnosis was reached and after 3 months the patient left on his own for Africa. On reviewing the history of this patient we found that he was interested in anthropology and that he had taken part in ritual interchange of blood with people belonging to remote tribes in East Africa ("blood brotherhood"). He had had a Tanzanian girlfriend when living in Tanzania.
>
> We believe that interchange of blood is a risk factor for AIDS equivalent to conventional exposure to blood and blood products... Although East Africa is not yet considered endemic with regard to AIDS, sexual transmission is another possible way that this patient acquired AIDS.
>
> The information we obtained from this patient while he was in our hospital illustrates the care that must be taken before risk factors are excluded in a patient with AIDS — especially if, as in this case, the patient

has impaired mental function due to toxoplasmosis and central-nervous-system lymphoma.[42]

No anthropological references were provided to support the patient's history of "blood brotherhood" ceremonies in remote tribes, and the authors themselves admit that the patient's mind was affected by his illness, and that there was no evidence of AIDS in East Africa at that time. Yet we are presented with the image of remote tribes infecting Europeans with their primitive rituals. The possibility that this sick man may have infected Africans is, of course, never considered. Such accounts always say more about European phantasies than African realities.

References
1. IC Bygbjerg. *AIDS in a Danish Surgeon (Zaire, 1976).* The Lancet, April 23, 1983, p925.
2. RJ Biggar, M Melbye, L Kestems et al. *Kaposi's sarcoma in Zaire not associated with HTLV-III Infection.* New England Journal of Medicine, Oct 18, 1984, Vol 311 No 16 p1051-2.
3. AC Bayley, R Chiengsong-Popov, AG Dalgliesh, RG Downing, RS Tedder, RA Weiss. *HTLV-III Serology Distinguishes Atypical and Endemic Kaposi's Sarcoma in Africa.* The Lancet, February 16 1985, p359-61.
4. AA Otu. *Kaposi's sarcoma and HTLV-III: a study in Nigerian adult males.* Journal of the Royal Society of Medicine, September 1986, Vol 79 p510-4
5. JA Levy, L-Z Pan, E Beth-Giraldo, LS Kaminsky et al. *Absence of antibodies of the human immunodeficiency virus in sera from Africa prior to 1975.* Proceedings of National Academy of Science USA, Medical Sciences, October 1986, Vol 83 p7935-37.
6. op cit AC Bayley, R Chiengsong-Popov et al
7. AC Bayley. *Aggressive Kaposi's sarcoma in Zambia, 1983.* The Lancet, June 16, 1984, p1318-20.
8. DIH Simpson. *The nasty viruses — Lassa, Marburg, and Ebola.* British Journal Hospital Medicine, February 1980, p191-4.
9. E Nnochiri. *Medical Microbiology in the Tropics.* Part Eleven, Systematic Virology, Oxford University Press, 1975, p265-309.
10. op cit IC Bygbjerg.
11. JW Curran. *AIDS — two years later.* New England Journal of Medicine, 1983, Vol 309 p609-11.
12. *Acquired Immune Deficiency Syndrome. Update: Evaluation of LAV/HTLV-III in health care personnel.* World Health Organisation, Weekly Epidemiological Record No 42, October 18, 1985.
13 Anonymous. *Needlestick transmission of HTLV-III from a patient infected in Africa.* The Lancet, December 15, 1984, p1376-7.

14. G Hunsmann, J Schneider, I Wendler, AF Fleming. *HTLV positivity in Africans.* The Lancet, October 26, 1985, Vol 2, p952-3.
15. I Wendler, J Schneider, B Gras, AF Fleming, G Hunsmann, H Schmitz. *Seroepidemiology of human immunodeficiency virus in Africa.* British Medical Journal, 27 September, 1986, Vol 293 p782-5.
16. op cit IC Bygbjerg.
17. W Sterry, M Marmor, A Konrads, GK Steigleder. *Kaposi's sarcoma, aplastic pancytopaenia, and multiple infections in a homosexual (Cologne, 1976).* The Lancet, April 23, 1983, p924.
18. J Vandepitte, R Verwilghen, P Zachee. *AIDS and Cryptococcosis (Zaire, 1977).* The Lancet, April 23, 1983, p925-6.
19. ibid J Vandepitte, R Verwilghen, P Zachee.
20. op cit JW Curran.
21. D Edwards, PG Harper, AK Pain et al. *Kaposi's sarcoma associated with AIDS in a woman from Uganda.* The Lancet, March 17, 1984, p631-2.
22. AEG Raine. EB Ilgren, JB Kurtz, JGG Ledingham, JA Waddell. *HTLV-III infection and AIDS in a Zambian nurse resident in Britain.* The Lancet, October 27, 1984, p985.
23. op cit AC Bayley, R Chiengsong-Popov et al.
24. P Jenkins, SR Malthouse, CA Banghan, JM Parkin, AJ Pinching. *AIDS: the African connection.* British Medical Journal, April 27, 1985, Vol 290 p1284-5.
25. ibid P Jenkins, SR Malthouse et al.
26. ibid P Jenkins, SR Malthouse et al.
27. LJ Eales, JM Parkin, SM Forster, KE Nye, JN Weber, JRW Harris, AJ Pinching. *Association of different forms of group specific component with susceptibility to and clinical manifestations of human immunodeficiency virus infection.* The Lancet, May 2, 1987, p999-1002.
28. D Vittecoq, J Modai. *AIDS in a black Malian.* The Lancet, October 29, 1983, p1023.
29. JB Brunet, J Chaperon, JC Gluckman et al. *Acquired immunodeficiency syndrome in France.* The Lancet, March 26, 1983, p700-1.
30. *Acquired immune deficiency syndrome (AIDS). Report on the situation in Europe as of 31 December 1984.* W.H.O. Weekly Epidemiological Record No 12, 22nd March 1985.
31. N Clumeck, F Mascart-Lemone, J de Maubeuge et al. *Acquired immunodeficiency syndrome in black Africans.* The Lancet, March 19, 1983, p642.
32. N Clumeck, J Sonnet, H Taelman, F Mascart-Lemone et al. *Acquired immunodeficiency syndrome in African patients.* New England Journal of Medicine, Feb 23, 1984, Vol 310 No 8 p492-7.
33. ibid N Clumeck, J Sonnet et al.
34. ibid N Clumeck, J Sonnet et al.
35. ibid N Clumeck, J Sonnet et al.
35. *Harrison's Principles of Internal Medicine.* 6th edition, McGraw-Hill Book Company, 1970, p875.
36. J Viera, E Frank, TJ Spira, SH Landesman. *Acquired Immune*

Deficiency in Haitians. New England Journal of Medicine, Jan 20, 1983, Vol 308 No 3 p125-9.

37. op cit N Clumeck, J Sonnet et al.
38. ibid N Clumeck, J Sonnet et al.
39. S Weissman. *The CIA and U.S. Policy in Zaire and Angola.* In *"Dirty Work: the CIA in Africa"*. Eds E Ray, W Schaap, K Van Meter and L Wolf, Zed Press, 1982, p157-81.
40. J Stockwell. *In Search of Enemies, A CIA Story.* Andre Deutsch, 1978.
41. op cit N Clumeck, J Sonnet et al.
42. L Morfeldt-Manson, L Lindquist. *Blood brotherhood: a risk factor for AIDS?* The Lancet, December 8, 1984, p1346.

Chapter 4

The New Scramble for Africa

In November 1983 the *British Medical Journal* published a review article titled "AIDS in Europe" by an American and two Danish doctors (R J Biggar, P Ebbersen and M Melbye) which intimated that AIDS had originated in Africa:

> A condition such as AIDS could have long existed in the African setting and gained entrance into America and Europe in recent years through increases in intercontinental travel. Only a definitive diagnostic test will permit us to be certain that the disease found in central Africa is a related phenomenon since it does not share the common epidemiological profile.[1]

The authors seriously attribute the appearance of AIDS in the United States in the late 1970's to a recent increase in intercontinental travel when at least ten million Africans had experienced a form of involuntary intercontinental travel in previous centuries.[2] Similar comments about a possible African origin of AIDS were made in other medical journals.[3,4]

These suggestions were formulated into a hypothesis by Dr Kevin de Cock who presented an article called "AIDS: an old disease from Africa?" in the *British Medical Journal* in August 1984. He summarised his ideas thus:

> It is suggested that the first Americans with AIDS acquired the condition in the early 1970's in Africa. AIDS is being increasingly recognized in Black Africans, and early African cases preceded the first documented American cases by several years...[5]

Dr de Cock offers an explanation for the transcontinental passage of the virus:

> The first American cases are likely to have become infected in the early

to mid-1970's, a time when tourism from the United States to Africa was developing as a result of heightened cultural interest.[6]

He seems quite undaunted by the fact that none of the early American cases were reported as giving any history of travel to Africa,[7] nor does he explain why the Americans were the first infected, rather than the French, British or Belgians whose colonial ties with central Africa would make them the most likely early candidates. The Americans with heightened cultural interest in Africa (in west and not central Africa) were black Americans stimulated by the novel "Roots", yet almost all the early American cases were white.[8]

Dr de Cock provides this explanation for the failure of physicians in Africa to diagnose AIDS prior to the American epidemic:

> In rural Africa diagnosis is often inexact. Fever is readily attributed to malaria without confirmation, and pneumonia is often assumed to be pneumococcal or tuberculous. Lack of facilities and the sheer volume of patients generally preclude more than basic investigation. Infections of all kinds are endemic and the major cause of death.[9]

For someone who worked in Kenya he displays an amazing ignorance of local conditions. Diagnostic facilities in rural areas are undoubtedly poor, but this is not the case in urban areas where teaching hospitals with good diagnostic facilities have been established for many years. There have been major shifts in population throughout the continent from rural to urban areas, voluntary and involuntary, for more than a century. Is it really conceivable that not a single victim of this chronic wasting disease ever left his village and found his way to hospital?

Dr de Cock further justifies his argument by raising the issue of Marburg and Lassa virus infections that were only identified when they infected white people,[10,11] and attributes the failure to identify these viruses in Africans to the poor diagnostic facilities. (The Marburg example is a complete red herring as only one natural infection has been reported, the remainder occurring in laboratory workers, and despite numerous endeavours no reservoir-host-vector chain has been found in animals or man anywhere in the world).[12] Earlier in the paper Dr de Cock stated that there was no evidence that any recently described infection has been caused by a genuinely new agent, and illustrated this point by referring to legionaire's disease and the toxic shock syndrome. The best western diagnostic facilities failed to identify these diseases that had previously existed in western countries until the recent outbreaks, yet Lassa fever and, by analogy, AIDS were not diagnosed in Africa because the facilities were poor. The arguments seem rather convenient. He then suggests that Africans are somehow better able to cope with AIDS than Europeans:

> The AIDS agent may exist in stable equilibrium with its rural African environment, but in a new population its expression may be altered by various factors including different innate susceptibility. Measles exemplifies this, being a generally mild infection that is nevertheless capable of decimating populations not previously exposed to it.[13]

We are told that Africans can somehow cope with the disease, but then again we are told that Africans, mostly from Zaire, began to seek treatment in Europe for AIDS-like illnesses in increasing numbers from 1977. Again, the case of the Danish surgeon and other early Zairean cases are uncritically accepted as evidence for a Zairean origin of the AIDS agent.

Dr de Cock then takes up the issue of Kaposi's sarcoma, a tumour associated with immune supression of various causes and a recurring theme in so many of the early papers on the African connection:

> As Kaposi's sarcoma was a feature in about one third of reported cases of AIDS, it would seem mandatory to look for AIDS where Kaposi's sarcoma has its highest incidence in the world, equatorial Africa....The relevance of Kaposi's sarcoma to AIDS is an important question, and it is surprising that the whole issue of the African tumour and its immunology has not received more attention.[14]

Without pausing for thought, he then discusses at length the restricted geographical location not just of Kaposi's sarcoma but a number of other tumours, including Burkitt's lymphoma, in the "lymphoma belt", 15 degrees north and south of the equator. To anyone capable of logical thought, the causative factor/s of any disease with a restricted geographical location will most probably be found in the environment, and these factors have not been ignored, but have been the substance of detailed research by eminent scientists such as Professor Burkitt. Let us remember that Dr de Cock, unlike many AIDS researchers in Africa, has a Diploma in Tropical Medicine and Hygiene. To quote from the standard textbook for the Diploma course, in this instance discussing Burkitt's lymphoma:

> It occurs in a geographical belt across Africa from east to west, within which the mean average temperature does not fall below 15.6 degrees Centigrade and the average rainfall is not less than 50 cm. The majority of cases have occurred in Africa and New Guinea... The exact cause is not known. Owing to the special geographical distribution of the tumour it has been suggested that a mosquito is responsible (Burkitt 1962) and that Anopheles spp. are the most likely, acting as vectors of an arthropod-bourne virus... and it is possible that malignant transformation following infection with the Epstein-Barr virus may take place against a

background of chronic lymphoreticular stimulation as the result of holoendemic malaria.[15]

Immune suppression is a well recognized complication of malaria infection.[16,17] There is no genetic predisposition for Kaposi's sarcoma, as people of African origin living outside the geographical area, for example black Americans and Caribbeans do not develop the tumour. No sexually transmitted disease has ever respected geography, and AIDS is certainly no exception. A proposal that HIV infection is responsible for Kaposi's sarcoma does not make scientific sense, and it is hardly surprising that numerous papers have been published that demonstrate no association between endemic KS and AIDS. For example a study of 37 adult Nigerian men with Kaposi's sarcoma concluded:

> Tropical African patients in the present study reproducibly failed to show anti-HTLV-III/LAV antibody. Endemic tropical KS and epidemic AIDS-linked KS seem to be two different diseases with possibly different aetiological agents.[18]

Mercifully, Dr de Cock concludes: "The arguments put forward are my own". His paper was met with wide acceptance and agreement, although some wished to add an individual contribution. Dr Peter Jones of the Newcastle Haemophilia Centre had pioneered the use of commercial American factor VIII in the United Kingdom. He disagreed with the suggestion that AIDS was introduced into America through sexual contact. He argued that in the 1970's major pharmaceutical companies regularly bought plasma from international plasma brokers who used cheap African and Haitian blood. He states:

> Given the long incubation period for AIDS these facts suggest that the disease was introduced into the United States not by sexual transmission but via plasma obtained in endemic areas. The exposure of a population with no natural resistance to the virus and with a proclivity for promiscuity resulted in spread.[19]

The pharmaceutical companies concerned denied using non-American products,[20] but in any case the arguments themselves do not stand up. If haemophiliacs, who are under continual medical supervision, were the initial western cases, this would have been very obvious in the early stages of the epidemic. Even by August 1983 only 15 of a total of 2008 cases (less than 1 per cent) of AIDS patients in the United States were haemophiliacs.

Dr de Cock called on scientists to prove his hypotheses:

> There is a need for international seroepidemiological studies of infection with HTLV-III and allied agents, including in African patients with AIDS and in areas in which Kaposi's sarcoma is endemic.[21]

Another scramble for Africa ensued.

In search of the rest of the "epidemiological iceberg" of AIDS cases, the scientists moved into central Africa. The Belgians spearheaded the expedition, but others were close behind. The Belgian effort was so well co-ordinated that the research by Dr.(now Professor) Piot's group in Zaire appeared in the same issue of *The Lancet* as those of Rouvroy, Van de Perre, Butzler and others who had set up camp in Rwanda.

Dr Piot in Zaire studied a total of 38 patients (20 males and 18 females) in the 3 weeks that their studies lasted. The patients were examined in the Mama Yemo and University hospitals in Kinshasa. They used the following definition for AIDS:

> ...an adult under 60 years of age who had evidence of an opportunistic infection or disseminated KS by histopathology, no underlying history of immunosupressive disease of immunosuppressive drug use, and who fulfilled two of the three immunological criteria of skin test anergy to multiple antigens, an absolute number of helper T lymphocytes (OKT 4) less than 400/ul. or a ratio of helper to suppressor T cells (OKT 4:OKT 8) less than 0.7. Opportunistic infections were defined as cryptococcal meningitis, cryptosporidiosis, extensive mucocutaneous herpes simplex virus (HSV) infection, bilateral pneumonia (by radiography) that was unresponsive to antibiotics or anti-tuberculous drugs, extensive oral/ oesophageal candidiasis, and chorioretinitis.[22]

These patients were compared with 26 controls, 12 of whom were suffering from infectious diseases. We then come to an extraordinary piece of science. Seven of the 13 controls with infectious diseases, including malaria and tuberculosis, had low helper-T cells and OKT 4/OKT 8 ratios. The authors themselves comment:

> Tuberculosis, protein calorie malnutrition, and various parasitic diseases can all be associated with depression of cellular immunity.[23]

In fact, pulmonary tuberculosis was suspected in 4 of these "AIDS" patients. Skin anergy, although not present in the controls, is a feature of patients with advanced tuberculosis, who are also prone to intercurrent opportunistic infections. The rate of malarial infection in Zaire is very high. Visceral leishmaniasis and African trypanosomiasis are also not uncommon. Surely, unless such diseases are carefully excluded, depressed cellular immunity would not support a diagnosis of AIDS. The authors are blissfully unaware of these contradictions:

> Because of limited diagnostic facilities we used a case definition which included clinical features of AIDS and the immunological characteristics of low T helper cell counts and low helper to suppressor ratios which have been the hallmarks of AIDS. We believe that this combination

strengthens the case definition in an area where severe infectious diseases abound, often going undiagnosed.[24]

On venturing into the field of epidemiology, our researchers make the following observation:

> 22 of the 38 cases were seen in hospitals which serve primarily private patients, a distinctly small proportion of the total population of Kinshasa. While rates of disease by socioeconomic status cannot yet be calculated these figures do suggest that a disproportionate number of cases may be occurring in the higher income population.[25]

This observation has been confirmed by many other subsequent studies. (Comparisons with the control group are meaningless as the patients were all drawn from the same hospitals). The researchers then perform a remarkable conjuring trick with statistics:

> Using as the numerator the number of cases of AIDS seen during the three weeks of this investigation and which came from Kinshasa and as a denominator the population of Kinshasa (about 3 million) we estimate the annual rate to be about 17 per 100,000. If children were excluded from the denominator the rate would be even higher. This is a minimal estimate, and it is comparable with or higher than the rate in San Francisco or New York.[26]

On the basis of a three week study, with limited diagnostic facilities, an unsound scientific method and a sample size of less than 30 patients, Kinshasa's AIDS problem is worse than San Francisco's!

How, then, did AIDS reach Zaire? Dr Piot and his team, like all other western researchers, seem quite unable to entertain the idea that the virus may have been introduced to Zaire from America or Europe, even though they present information that strongly suggests such a possibility. In the paper they discuss two clusters of AIDS in heterosexual partners in Kinshasa, many of whom had been diagnosed in Belgium. AIDS, it would seem, is a disease of promiscuous Africans of high socio-economic status who travel abroad, surely the very people to acquire and import a new disease. Even at the time of the paper's publication it was generally accepted that AIDS was an unwelcome American import into Haiti,[27] so why not Zaire? Of all the black African states, Zaire has the closest political and military links with the United States. Kinshasa alone has over 200,000 expatriates, forming 8% of its population.[28] Recently an American who worked in Zaire successfully sued his company for worker's compensation because he claimed he had contracted AIDS from prostitutes procured by the company for "recreational sex".[29] Our own interviews with expatriates from Zaire confirmed widespread sexual exploitation of the Zairean population, both homosexual and heterosexual. As in Haiti, there are very strong taboos against homosexuality in most African countries, and homosexual Africans (many of whom are bisexual) are very unlikely to admit their sexual preferences. But minds convinced of an African origin are unable to explore such possibilities.

In a four week period in Kigali, Rwanda, Phillipe Van de Perre, Dominique Rouvroy *et al* diagnosed 26 patients (17 males and 9 females). These patients were selected in a similar manner to those in Zaire. They summarised their findings as follows:

> 16 patients had opportunistic infections, associated with KS in only 2; 1 had multifocal KS alone; and 9 had clinical conditions consistent with prodrome of AIDS. All patients had severe T-cell defects characterised by cutaneous anergy, a striking decrease in the number of helper T-cells, and a decreased OKT4:OKT8 ratio.[30]

The limited presentation of the clinical findings in this paper precludes a detailed review. Four patients classified as AIDS and three patients with the AIDS prodrome (ie with lymphadenopathy, weight loss and diarrhoea) had tuberculosis. The white blood cell count may be low in disseminated tuberculosis, and T-cell abnormalities would not just support a diagnosis of AIDS.[31] Another "AIDS" patient had an amoebic liver abcess, not a recognized association with AIDS. Salmonella septicaemia was found in two cases, and diarrhoea, fever and weight loss in these patients would not necessarily indicate AIDS. A child with interstitial pneumonia included in the series was only considered a probable case of AIDS by the authors. The ocular findings reported in one patient with disseminated tuberculosis and another with cryptococcal septicaemia are entirely consistent with the primary diagnosis and do not imply an additional cytomegalovirus infection. One male patient had multifocal KS (lymph nodes and skin alone). The authors themselves comment that T-cell defects are associated with endemic KS, an entity they consider probably unrelated to AIDS. One is left wondering how many of these cases were genuinely AIDS. The Belgian doctors themselves had no such doubts:

> In most developing countries body scanning, brain biopsy, and bronchoalveolar lavage are impracticable. Few opportunistic infections are easy to demonstrate. The results reported here may thus underestimate the true pattern of opportunistic infections in African patients.[32]

The Rwandan team reached similar epidemiological conclusions to their colleagues in Zaire:

> This study confirms that AIDS exists in Rwanda, a central African country ᴖast of Zaire. The detection of 26 AIDS patients in a short period suggests

that AIDS may be a public health problem in central Africa... From mid-1983 cases of oesophageal candidiasis increased sharply. The increasing incidence of oesophageal candidiasis and our estimate of the annual incidence of AIDS (80 cases per 100,000 in Kigali) suggest that AIDS could be endemic in urban areas of central Africa...[33]

The figure of 80 per 100,000 was arrived at using the now familiar statistical method of the Belgians. They conclude:

The African patients with AIDS reported in Belgium were of high socioeconomic status. These data could have been biased by the fact that only the privileged patients could afford to travel to Europe for medical care. However, many patients in our Rwandan series were also relatively well-to-do. Most of them were town based professionals working in the private or public sectors. Although the 1978 census showed that more than 93% of the Rwandan population is rural, the patients reported here belonged to the minority of people in contact with Kigali and the chief towns and prefectures. Urban activity, a reasonable standard of living, heterosexual promiscuity, and contacts with prostitutes could be risk factors for African AIDS...[34]

Let us remind ourselves that European researchers became interested in Africa because they believed there was an association between AIDS and African Kaposi's sarcoma, and they had found a few cases of AIDS in Africans in Europe. Instead of finding the rest of the epidemiological "iceberg", they found a disease concentrated in the wealthy elite, epidemics of opportunistic infections that began in Zaire in 1981 and Rwanda in 1983, and they could find no link between KS and their AIDS cases. The evidence was pointing to a disease introduced from abroad, although inevitably this was not the European's perception.

References

1. P Ebbesen, RJ Biggar, M Melbye. *AIDS in Europe.* British Medical Journal, November 5, 1983, Vol 287 p1324-6.
2. B Davidson. *Africa in History.* Granada Publishing Limited, 1978, p207.
3. IC Bygbjerg. *AIDS in a Danish surgeon.* The Lancet, April 23, 1983, p925.
4. N Clumeck, J Sonnet, H Taelman et al. *Acquired immunodeficiency syndrome in African patients.* New England Journal of Medicine, 1984, Vol 310 p492-7.
5. KM de Cock. *AIDS: an old disease from Africa?* British Medical Journal, August 4, 1984, Vol 289 p306-8.
6. ibid KM de Cock.
7. SM Freidman, YM Felman, R Rothenberg et al. *Follow-up on Kaposi's sarcoma and Pneumocystis pneumonia.* Morbidity and Mortality Weekly Report, August 28, 1981, Vol 30 No 33 p409-10.

8. ibid SM Freidman, YM Felman et al.
9. op cit KM de Cock.
10. EE Vella. *Marburg virus disease.* Hospital Update, January 1977, p35-41.
11. FA Murphy. *Marburg and Ebola Viruses.* In *Virology.* Eds BN Fields et al. Raven Press, New York, 1985.
12. op cit EE Vella.
13. op cit KM de Cock.
14. ibid KM de Cock.
15. C Wilcocks, PEC Manson-Bahr. *Manson's Tropical Diseases.* Bailliere Tindall, 1972, p14-5.
16. op cit N Clumeck, J Sonnet, H Taelman et al.
17. SD Dube, KR Krishnamurthy, S Baskarnathan. *Case report A case of disseminated Cryptococcosis.* Central African Journal of Medicine, July 1984, Vol 30 No 7 p120-3.
18. AA Otu. *Kaposi's sarcoma and HTLV-III: a study in Nigerian adult males.* Journal of the Royal Society of Medicine, September 1986, Vol 79 p510-4.
19. P Jones. *AIDS: the African connection?* British Medical Journal, March 23, 1985, Vol 290 p932.
20. C McAuley. *AIDS: the African connection?* British Medical Journal, May 18, 1985, Vol 290 p1517.
21. op cit KM de Cock.
22. P Piot, H Taelman, KB Minlange et al. *Acquired immunodeficiency syndrome in a heterosexual populatin in Zaire.* The Lancet, July 14, 1984, p65-9.
23. ibid P Piot, H Taelman, KB Minlange et al.
24. ibid P Piot, H Taelman, KB Minlange et al.
25. ibid P Piot, H Taelman, KB Minlange et al.
26. ibid P Piot, H Taelman, KB Minlange et al.
27. J Viera, E Frank, TJ Spira, SH Landesman. *Acquired Immune Deficiency Syndrome in Haitians.* New England Journal of Medicine, Jan 20, 1983, Vol 308 No 3 p125-9.
28. *West Africa*, March 2, 1987, p443.
29. *The Guardian*, March 6, 1987
30. P Van de Perre, P Lepage, P Kestelyn et al. *Acquired immunodeficiency syndrome in Rwanda.* The Lancet, July 14, 1984, p62-5.
31. *Harrison's Principles of Internal Medicine.* 6th edition, McGraw-Hill Book Company, 1970, p875.
32. op cit P Van de Perre, P Lepage, P Kestelyn et al.
33. ibid P Van de Perre, P Lepage, P Kestelyn et al.
34. ibid P Van de Perre, P Lepage, P Kestelyn et al.

Chapter 5

Problems of Diagnosis

The reliability of the diagnosis of AIDS in Haitian and African patients has been questioned by doctors who have argued that the symptoms and signs of a number of diseases common in the tropics may have been confused with those of AIDS.[1,2,] We would like to examine this issue in a little detail.

When a doctor examines a patient, he/she will firstly take a history of the illness, enquiring about the nature of the symptoms, time of onset, their severity and duration and so on. This is followed by an examination searching for physical signs of disease. The doctor can then formulate a provisional diagnosis that may include a number of different diseases that could account for the clinical findings. Sometimes the symptoms and signs alone are sufficient for a conclusive diagnosis, but frequently further investigations such as blood tests and x-rays are required before a definitive diagnosis can be reached.[3]

AIDS was first recognized when a number of young and previously healthy men died of pneumonia caused by *Pneumocystis carinii*.[4] This infection is rare in healthy people as the organism is not very pathogenic ie it is readily destroyed by the body's immune system, but it is more common in people whose immune system is damaged in some way, for example by leukaemia, a disorder of the white blood cells that fight infection, or by immunosuppressive drugs given to organ transplant patients to prevent rejection. Further investigation of the patients with pneumocystis pneumonia revealed that they had a reduced number of T-helper cells, white blood cells responsible for fighting certain types of infection. It was clear that the immune system of these patients was damaged by an unknown cause, so the disease was called the Acquired Immune Deficiency Syndrome.

The term "syndrome" is defined in *Harrison's Textbook of Internal Medicine* in the following way:

> ...a group of symptoms and signs of disorders of somatic (ie bodily) function, related to one another by means of some anatomic, physiologic, or biochemical peculiarity of the organism. It embodies a hypothesis concerning the deranged function of an organ, organ system or tissue....A syndromic diagnosis usually does not indicate the precise cause of an illness, but it greatly narrows the number of possibilities and, thus, suggests whatever further clinical and laboratory studies are required.[5]

The causative organism, the human immunodeficiency virus (HIV), previously termed HTLV-III/LAV, was not identified until two years after AIDS was first recognized.[6] Although AIDS is now widely accepted as the name of the disease, it is a syndromic diagnosis, and would now be more accurately termed something like human immunodeficiency virus disease.

As the human immunodeficiency virus is not the only cause of disorders of the immune system and a number of other diseases can present with symptoms and signs similar to AIDS, a diagnosis of AIDS on clinical and laboratory evidence of opportunistic diseases can be inaccurate unless it is confirmed by reliable tests for actual infection with the virus. These problems can be compounded by the well known phenomenon of observer bias. The following comment is made in *Harrison's* text:

> The physician does not start with an open mind any more than does the scientist, but with one prejudiced from knowledge of recent cases; and the patient's first statement directs his thinking in certain channels. He must struggle constantly to avoid the bias occasioned by his own attitude, mood, irritability, and interest.[7]

The pattern of disease varies greatly in different human communities, determined by such factors as standards of nutrition, housing and sanitation, and the various infectious agents that inhabit different geographical locations.[8] For example many insect vectors such as the mosquitoes that transmit malaria only live in warm climates, and tuberculosis occurs most commonly in areas where poor nutrition and overcrowding prevail.[9] Thus chronic wasting diseases such as advanced tuberculosis that may be clinically similar to AIDS are uncommon in well nourished and well housed white American communities, but are endemic in poor immigrant Haitians.[10] A number of diseases that occur in tropical countries, including visceral leishmaniasis (Kala Azar) and African trypanosomiasis (sleeping sickness) present with fever, weight loss, skin rashes and lymphadenopathy, common symptoms of AIDS, and sufferers frequently die of intercurrent opportunistic diseases.[11] Suppression of the immune system that can be induced by parasitic diseases and malnutrition can add to the diagnostic difficulties.[12] Familiarity with the pattern of disease in a community is essential for a high degree of diagnostic accuracy, and many doctors who have practised medicine in temperate, industrialised countries experience great initial difficulty in recognizing diseases in rural communities in tropical climates. American and European doctors, prejudiced from recent experience of cases of AIDS in their own countries and unfamiliar with tropical diseases could, without too much difficulty, reach the wrong diagnostic conclusions.

The circumstances mentioned above may not be the only explanation for possible misdiagnosis of AIDS in black people, whether Haitian or African. There is no reason to believe that doctors are immune from the racism that is such an integral part of western culture, and indeed the medical text books and journals are littered with examples of classic racist thought. We can cite many examples, but will limit ourselves to two:

> ...hypermetropia (long-sightedness), while it is physiological in children, represents from the biological stand-point an imperfectly developed eye when it persists into adult life. Most primitive peoples and many of the lower animals are hypermetropic; carnivora, for example, are almost constantly so.[13]

There is, of course, no scientific basis for this statement. An item on race and diet can be found in one of the standard textbooks for general surgery, by Bailey and Love:

> Appendicitis is particularly common in the highly civilised European, American, and Australasian countries, while it is rare in Asiatics, Africans, and Polynesians. Rendle Short showed that if individuals from the latter races migrate to the countries where appendicitis is common, they soon acquire the local susceptibility to the disease. Even apes in captivity appear to acquire the human liability to appendicitis. These significant facts satisfy many that the rise in appendicitis amongst the highly civilised is due to a departure from a simple diet rich in cellulose to one relatively rich in meat.[14]

Clearly appendicitis has nothing to do with race or civilisation, unless the acquisition of a less healthy diet is a hallmark of civilisation. And do we civilise primates when we put them in cages? Surgeons in East Africa joked that their patients did not develop appendicitis until they learned to speak English. The racial obsessions of the doctors and medical researchers are discussed elsewhere in the book, but suffice it to say here that racist associations of black people with disease, dirt and excessive sexuality may have influenced the researchers to overdiagnose AIDS in black people and attribute them with its source.

Let us consider some of the diseases that may be confused with AIDS by the unwary western doctor. Tuberculosis is now a relatively uncommon disease in industrialised societies but remains very common in the Third World.[15] Tuberculous infection confined to the lungs can be diagnosed without too much difficulty, but if the tubercle bacillis gains access to the blood stream diagnosis may be extremely difficult even in hospitals with good diagnostic facilities. The clinical features of massive disseminated (miliary) tuberculosis are described in the following way:

> Symptoms are usually nonspecific and consist of weight loss, weakness, gastrointestinal disturbances, fever, and sweats... Cough is not a prominent feature, but dyspnea (shortness of breath) may be. The correct diagnosis is often not suspected until the typical "miliary" pattern appears on the roentgenogram (X-ray) of the lungs. The white blood count may be normal or low, or may show a leukemoid pattern. One useful feature of the blood count is the finding of a decreased ratio of lymphocytes to monocytes (normal 3:1).[16]

Subacute and chronic forms of haematogenous tuberculosis are also described, and, according to *Harrison's* textbook, occur at a younger age in black people than in whites:

> (There are) a variety of clinical manifestations including aplastic anaemia, low-grade fever, lymphadenopathy....This clinical picture is most common among Negroes of any age and in Caucasians of advanced years, and the process represents an overwhelming of immunity during reactivation of tuberculosis after years of dormancy. The protean manifestations and bizarre clinical pictures....provide a tremendous diagnostic challenge. To add to the confusion, the tuberculin reaction is often suppressed in persons with overwhelming infection.[17]

The similarity between the clinical presentation of AIDS and haematogenous tuberculosis can easily lead to misdiagnosis, a similarity that extends to the reduced white cell count and the absence of a tuberculin reaction. Several researchers comment on the high incidence of tuberculosis in Haitian and African AIDS patients.[18,19,20] Diagnostic confusion seems a distinct possibility.

Visceral leishmaniasis is another disease that may be easily confused with AIDS. A letter was published in the Transactions of the Royal Society of Tropical Medicine and Hygiene (1985) titled "Leishmaniasis or AIDS?":

> The recent description of the acquired immunodeficiency syndrome (AIDS) has had a great psychosocial impact. However its correct diagnosis

remains difficult. We present here a case which posed serious doubts in diagnosis...

A 20 year-old heterosexual man with type A haemophilia, who had been treated with factor VIII concentrates, was admitted to hospital in April 1983 with a history of several months of fever and diarrhoea...While in hospital, chest X-rays revealed two episodes of bronchopneumonia.

In July 1983, persistent cough, weight loss, general malaise and minimal hepatosplenomegaly were added to his initial symptoms... *Candida albicans* was isolated from the oral mucosa, faeces and urine, and was treated with ketoconazole. Leukopaenia was noted..., as well as anaemia... A sternal bone marrow puncture revealed few cells, a decrease in helper T lymphocytes... and an inverted helper/suppressor ratio. Hepatosplenomegaly increased from July to September, and generalised lymphadenopathy was noted for several days. A second bone marrow puncture performed on 6th September showed Leishmania....

Retrospective serological studies... confirmed *L. donovani* infection was present several months before the diagnosis was made. Until then we strongly suspected a case of pre-AIDS... For these reasons, we would like to point out the need to exclude the possibility of *L. donovani* infection in all patients with cellular immunodeficiency in countries with visceral leishmaniasis or in those who have visited such countries.[21]

Visceral leishmaniasis occurs in all the central and east African countries[22] where AIDS is said to have reached epidemic proportions.

An illustration of the probable misdiagnosis of cases of AIDS in African patients is the case of the drug Suramin. This drug has been used to treat a number of tropical diseases including onchocerciasis and trypanosomiasis.[23] A group of Belgian doctors who had been eagerly diagnosing AIDS in Rwanda treated five patients with the drug:

All five patients (with AIDS-related complex) had fever, night sweats, loss of more than 10% body weight lasting for 5-12 months, and oesophageal candidiasis. Other symptoms included generalised lymphadenopathy, chronic diarrhoea, and chronic arthralgias...

All patients improved after the first injection of suramin. The lymphadenopathy, arthralgias, and diarrhoea disappeared... OKT4 lymphocytes and OKT4/OKT8 ratio rose in four patients. Delayed hypersensitivity reaction to tuberculin and PHA was restored in three patients tested but remained negative for candidin.

This preliminary study suggests that suramin influenced the short-term clinical and immunological progress of four of these five patients...[24]

Suramin was then given to ten white American patients with acquired immunodeficiency syndrome presenting as Kaposi's sarcoma or AIDS-related complex. The detectable virus level fell in four patients in whom virus was isolated prior to therapy. The authors conclude:

Despite this in-vivo virustatic effect, no significant clinical or immunological improvement was observed using this short-term regimen.[25]

West German doctors tried the drug on eight patients with AIDS-related complex or AIDS, one of whom was an African.[26] Only the African showed any improvement, and the authors suggested that Africans in general tolerate suramin better than Europeans. The thought that they may have been treating tropical diseases such as African trypanosomiasis that are clinically similar to AIDS does not seem to have crossed their minds.

Further evidence that AIDS may have been overdiagnosed in Africans can be inferred from the World Health Organisation statistics. If we look at the number of new cases of AIDS diagnosed in Europe since 1984, the figures have been doubling approximately every twelve months, yet during this period the number of African cases diagnosed in Europe has actually been declining.[27]

New AIDS cases reported in Europe

	Africans	Total
1984 (April to Dec)	84	477
1985 (Jan to Dec)	64	1244
1986 (Jan to Dec)	53	2543

Interestingly the same phenomenon occurred in Haitians in the United States.[28] The Belgians attributed the decrease in Zairean new cases to the setting up of facilities for treating these patients in Zaire,[29] a rather odd claim when we consider the ineffectiveness of treatment anywhere in the world. In any case two-thirds of the African patients developed the disease whilst resident in Europe. The genuine explanation for the decline in African cases may be the introduction of reliable blood tests for AIDS antibodies in late 1984/early 1985 that would have largely eliminated the diagnostic confusion between AIDS and other diseases.

References
1. JW Mellors, M Barry. *Malnutrition or AIDS in Haiti?* New England Journal of Medicine, April 26, 1984, Vol 310 No 17 p1119-1120.
2. Y Adeyemi. *The origin of AIDS.* Concord Weekly, July 11, 1985, p46.
3. *Harrison's Principles of Internal Medicine, Chapter 2, Approach to Disease.* McGraw-Hill, 1970, p4-7.

4. MS Gottlieb, HM Shanker, PT Fan et al. *Pneumocystis pneumonia — Los Angeles*. Morbidity and Mortality Weekly Report, June 5, 1981, Vol 30 No 21 p250-1.
5. op cit *Harrison's Principles of Internal Medicine*, p6.
6. F Barre-Sinoussi, JC Cheerman, F Rey et al. *Isolation of a T-lymphotrophic retrovirus from a patient at risk for acquired immune deficiency syndrome (AIDS)*. Science, 1983, Vol 220, p868-70.
7. op cit *Harrison's Principles of Internal Medicine*, p6.
8. AO Lucas, HM Giles. *A short textbook of preventive mecicine in the tropics*. The English Universities Press, 1973, p1-3.
9. ibid AO Lucas, HM Giles, p221-7.
10. J Viera, E Frank, T Spira et al. *Acquired Immune Deficiency in Haitians*. New England Journal of Medicine, Jan 20 1983, Vol 308 No 3, p125-9
11. C Wilcocks, PEC Manson-Bahr. *Manson's Tropical Diseases*. Bailliere Tindall, 1974, pp98 and 124.
12. N Clùmeck, J Sonnet, H Taelman et al. *Acquired immunodeficiency syndrome in African patients*. New England Journal of Medicine, February 23, 1984, Vol 310 No 8, p492-7.
13. D Abrams. *Duke-Elder's Practice of Refraction*. Churchill Livingstone, 1978, p37.
14. *Bailey and Love's Short Practice of Surgery*, 17th edition, revised by AJ Harding-Rains and H David Ritchie, HK Lewis and Co. Ltd, London, 1977, p1027.
15. op cit *Manson's Tropical Diseases*, p447.
16. op cit *Harrison's Principles of Internal Medicine*, p875.
17. ibid *Harrison's Principles of Internal Medicine*, p875.
18. op cit J Viera, E Frank, T Spira et al.
19. P Piot, H Taelman, KB Minlange et al. *Acquired immunodeficiency syndrome in a heterosexual population in Zaire*. The Lancet, July 14, 1984, p65-9.
20. P Van de Perre, P Lepage, P Kestelyn et al. *Acquired immunodeficiency syndrome in Rwanda*. The Lancet, July 14, 1984, p62-5.
21. A de la Loma, J Alvar, E Martinez Galiano et al. *Leishmaniasis or AIDS?* Transactions of the Royal Society of Tropical Medicine and Hygiene, 1985, Vol 79 p421-2.
22. op cit *Manson's Tropical Diseases*, p117-32.
23. ibid *Manson's Tropical Diseases*, pp102 and 234.
24. D Rouvroy, J Bogaerts, J-B Habyarimana et al. *Short-term results with suramin for AIDS-related conditions*. The Lancet, April 13, 1985, p878-9.
25. S Broder, JM Collins, PD Markham, RC Gallo et al. *Effects of suramin on HTLV-III/LAV infection presenting as Kaposi's sarcoma or AIDS-related complex: clinical pharmacology and suppression of virus replication in vivo*. The Lancet, September 21, 1985, p627-30.
26. W Busch, R Brodt, A Ganser et al. *Suramin treatment for AIDS*. The Lancet, November 30, 1985, p1247.
27. These figures are derived from the following WHO Weekly Epidemiological Records, *Acquired Immunodeficiency Syndrome (AIDS):* No 32,

August 10, 1984, p249-50; No 40, October 5, 1984, p305-7; No 12, March 22, 1985, p85-90; No 25, June 21, 1985, p189-90; No 40, October 4, 1985, p305-11; No 2, January 10, 1986, p5-7; No 17, April 25, 1986, p125-8; No 28, July 11, 1986, p213-4; No 40, October 3, 1986, p305-6; No 5, January 30, 1987, p23-5; No 17, April 24, 1987, p117-21.

28. KM de Cock. *AIDS: an old disease from Africa?* British Medical Journal, August 4, 1984, Vol 289 p306-8.

29. *Acquired immunodeficiency syndrome (AIDS). Report on the situation in Europe as of 31 December 1984.* WHO Weekly Epidemiological Record No 12, March 22, 1985, p85-90.

Chapter 6

Seroepidemiology

Evidence for a recent onset of AIDS in central Africa was provided by Ann Bayley, Professor of Surgery at the University Teaching Hospital, Lusaka, Zambia. Records had been kept for many years of all patients in Lusaka who developed Kaposi's sarcoma, and until 1983 the clinical presentation and tumour behaviour conformed to descriptions of endemic KS. In 1983 she noticed a change:

> 10 men, mean age 41, presented with typical symptoms and signs (nodules or plaques on oedematous limbs, with florid tumours or woody infiltration) and all 10 patients responded promptly to actinomycin D and vincristine. 13 patients (10 men and 3 women), mean age 27, presented with unusual symptoms and signs, including generalised lesions, respiratory distress, gross weight loss, and absence of nodules and plaques on the limbs. 8 of 13 patients with atypical KS failed to maintain an initial response to chemotherapy and died before the end of 1983, but there were no deaths amongst patients with endemic disease.[1]

Two men admitted to single episodes of homosexual behaviour, but both said this had occurred after the onset of symptoms of KS. There were epidemiological differences between the patients with classical and atypical KS:

> Patients with atypical disease were younger than those with classical KS, and they were better educated and had better jobs; 4 had the same professional background, suggesting an occupational or social cluster.[2]

Doctors in Africa were clearly able to recognize a new phenomenon, and support for the "Old Disease" hypothesis could not be substantiated. But for those diehards who wished to believe that Africa had infected the world, a wonderful new tool was placed in their hands.

After the virus was isolated in 1983 blood tests for AIDS antibodies could be developed, and these became available in 1984. Researchers spread themselves across central Africa collecting blood from all and sundry, and delved into the bottom of their freezers for blood specimens collected on previous safaris. They came up with some startling results. Robert Biggar, Mads Melbye and others went to rural Zaire:

In May 1984, 250 outpatients at a hospital in a remote area of eastern Zaire were surveyed for AIDS type illnesses and the prevalence of antibodies against HTLV-III determined by an enzyme linked immunosorbent assay using disrupted whole HTLV-III virus as the antigen. No clinical cases of AIDS were diagnosed among these patients. Overall, 31 (12.4%) had clearly positive ratios ($\geq$5.0) and a further 30 (12.0%) had borderline ratios (3.0-<5.0). Western blots of serum samples from subjects with antibodies yielded bands consistent with HTLV-III as found in American patients with AIDS and members of groups at risk of AIDS. The prevalence of antibody was highest in childhood (p=0.02); among adults prevalence rose slightly with age. HTLV-III antibodies were more common among the uneducated (p=0.006), agricultural workers (p=0.03), and rural residents (p=0.06), but the Western blot bands were generally weak in this group. By contrast, one urban resident had strong bands.

The relatively high prevalence of antibodies among the rural poor in this area of Zaire suggests that HTLV-III or a closely related, cross reactive virus may be endemic in the region. A different natural history of infection, perhaps in childhood, may also explain the findings.[3]

Here was an extraordinary situation. Nearly a quarter of a poor, rural population had some evidence of exposure to the virus, yet the only Zaireans who had developed the disease were from the wealthy, well educated elite resident in the cities. The authors offered a number of explanations for this contradiction:

There are several possible explanations. The greater prevalence of HTLV-III among children in this study might support a hypothesis in which the adult population has been exposed to HTLV-III infection in childhood, with some of the children who were infected being lost from the study population. An extension would be that the influx of an infected rural population (adapted biologically to the virus) into an urban area with a pool of susceptible, more affluent adults created new opportunities for the virus to cause illness in urban adults and the epidemic appearance of the disease in Africa...

The possibility of non-specific results must be considered, since a high frequency of non-confirmed ELISA positivity against a related human retrovirus, HTLV-I, was found in subjects from Ghana, west Africa. Nevertheless, the correlation between Western blotting and ELISA results for HTLV-III in this study was excellent... This reactivity suggests that the provoking agent was HTLV-III or a highly cross reactive virus.

With regard to the latter possibility, the assay may be measuring responses to a similar and cross reactive virus that does not have the pathogenicity of the AIDS related HTLV-III. Such a virus might be the ancestor from which a new variant, pathogenic AIDS related HTLV-III, has recently mutated, or it might be another new member of the family of retroviruses...[4]

A new twist was added to the "Old Disease of Africa" hypothesis. The virus was in darkest Africa all along, but just happened to mutate, find its way to the cities, and from there to the west coast of America, bypassing the more likely routes through Europe on the way.

Even more startling were the findings which emerged from a study conducted in Kenya by 12 researchers including Robert Biggar and Robert C. Gallo. Overall, 21% of the population studied were seropositive, but in one ethnic group, the Turkana, 50% were positive. Still, there were no cases of AIDS:

In view of the high prevalence of HTLV-III antibody, AIDS illness might have been expected to be frequent, yet no cases have been documented in Kenya. We are aware of only three cases suspected of being AIDS-related in Kenya. All were diagnosed in Nairobi... Given the quality of medical care available in Kenya, it is unlikely that AIDS-illnesses of the recognized varieties are occurring at a rate commensurate with the prevalence of antibody against HTLV-III.[5]

The authors themselves express some doubts about their findings:

One common link may be the presence of chronic parasitemia. In Ghana, West Africa, ELISA antibody against HTLV-I was found more frequently in subjects with a high titre of antibody against malaria.[6]

They also noted that patients with splenomegaly (enlarged spleen) had a high incidence of seropositivity, and speculated that this may have been due to HTLV-III infection, as mice with a related retrovirus infection also developed splenomegaly. This is all rather obscure. By far the commonest cause of splenomegaly in the tropics is chronic malarial infection, which is also responsible for false positivity of an ELISA test for a similar virus. Were our researchers merely identifying malaria, and not AIDS?

Researchers delved even deeper into their deep freezers and produced blood collected in Uganda in 1972, publishing their results in a paper titled "Evidence for exposure to HTLV-III in Uganda before 1973". The blood was collected as part of a study of Burkitt's lymphoma, a tumour that is associated with malaria. The mean age

of the patient population was 6.4 years, and an overall positive rate
of 66% was found. The authors experienced a now familiar problem:

> ...our samples were taken from a sparsely populated subsistence-farming
> environment where AIDS is not known to occur, while the recent spread
> in African AIDS appears to be in more densely populated urban
> environments and heterosexual populations.[7]

But they explained away these difficulties with the usual arguments:

> If, as we suspect, the antibody reactivities found represent widespread
> exposure or infection by HTLV-III, then it must be asked why the
> incidence of AIDS in the Ugandan population (and neighbouring Zaire)
> has gone unnoticed for so long. It is possible that AIDS existed in African
> populations without being recognized as a separate disease entity. The
> virus may have originated in Africa in the past, and exposure to the virus
> may be more common than AIDS itself in some populations.[8]

Let us remember that the blood samples were collected by a team
of researchers studying an opportunistic tumour, Burkitt's lymphoma,
in a country where eminent scientists such as Professor Burkitt had
carried out extensive research for many years. It is hard to believe
that AIDS, if present in this community, would not have been
recognized as a clinical entity.

One of the papers most widely quoted to support an African origin
for AIDS was published as a letter to *The Lancet* in May 1986:

> The place of origin of HTLV-III is controversial but most workers have
> suggested Africa. Most cogent to the issue has been the isolation of a
> related virus from the African green monkey, the high incidence of AIDS
> in many central African countries, and serological evidence for a high
> prevalence of infection. Because of the importance of this issue we
> decided to test 1213 plasmas, obtained originally for immunogenetic
> studies, from various parts of Africa, of which 818 had been obtained as
> far back as 1959. We appreciate that enzyme immunoassay antibody tests
> on sera or plasma frozen for many years can lead to false-positive
> results...[9]

Blood was collected from groups of people categorised as: 1967
Mozambique; rural Bantu, 1982 Congo; rural bantu — terms even
the South Africans now avoid. Only one specimen was positive:

> We have demonstrated that at least 1 individual from central Africa had
> been exposed to a virus similar to human HTLV-III more than a quarter
> of a century ago. The identity of the donor is no longer known. Our results
> also suggest that the prevalence of HTLV-III was very low in central
> Africa in 1959.[10]

Firstly the authors stated that tests on plasma frozen for many years
can give false positive results, secondly only one of 1213 specimens

was positive, and thirdly the authors are not even convinced that the individual had actually been exposed to HTLV-III. Yet this much quoted paper proved that AIDS originated in Zaire!

The doubts about the reliability of a blood test that found widespread AIDS virus infection in communities with no clinical cases of AIDS could not be ignored. Robert Biggar and co-workers investigated several seropositive Zairean subjects without clinical AIDS and found no evidence of immune deficiency.[11] They rechecked the blood samples they had collected in rural Zaire for antibodies against the commonest form of malaria, *Plasmodium falciparum*, publishing their results in *The Lancet* in September 1985:

> A serological survey of 250 outpatients in rural Zaire showed that the prevalence of antibody against HTLV-I, HTLV-II, and HTLV-III, as detected by enzyme-linked immunosorbent assay, correlated strongly with level of antibodies against *Plasmodium falciparum*. The age curve for the prevalence of antibody against these retroviruses and high titres of antibodies against *P. falciparum* were similar.[12]

The authors offered several possible explanations for these findings:

> 1. Infection with malaria and all three HTLV retroviruses could be unrelated but share similar environmental factors such as those related to increasing age and rural poverty... 2. The human retroviruses could be transmitted by mosquitoes or within the parasite itself... 3. Malaria and other parasitic diseases could act indirectly by influencing host immune response...[13]

Contrast this with the Belgian researchers' claim that African AIDS patients were relatively affluent and came from an urban environment,[14,15] where the incidence of malaria is lower than in the rural areas. The fourth proposal seems by far the most likely:

> 4. Finally, reactivity in both ELISA and western blot analysis may be non-specific in healthy Africans... If the human retrovirus reactivity observed in the ELISA test is frequently non-specific among Africans, the causes of the non-specificity need to be clarified in order to determine how they might affect the seroepidemiology of retroviruses in areas other than Africa, such as the Caribbean and Japan. Serological studies from Africa would also need to be re-evaluated with a more specific test before conclusions can be drawn.[16]

More specific tests, for example the indirect immunofluorescence, were available in 1985, and serious scientists would surely have rechecked at least a proportion of their positive results. Inevitably conclusions were drawn and there was a lot of informed opinion that announced to the ever gullible world that mosquitoes were spreading AIDS in Africa.

False-positivity was emerging as a problem not just in Africa, but in the United States itself. The *New England Journal of Medicine* published a letter in January 1986 titled "Asymptomatic Blood Donor with a False Positive HTLV-III Western Blot":

> The patient was a 34-year-old woman from rural Alabama who donated blood in May 1985. Initial testing at the local blood bank revealed that she was positive for HTLV-III antibody by ELISA tests on two separate occasions. Her serum was sent for verification to the designated commercial laboratory, where three repeat ELISAs were strongly positive..., as was the Western blot assay... In July 1985, the patient was informed that her serum was positive for HTLV-III antibody.
>
> On clinical examination the patient was anxious but otherwise asymptomatic. Her physical examination was normal. Both she and her husband of 14 years denied any homosexual or extramarital sexual encounters, intravenous drug abuse, blood transfusions, or foreign travel...
>
> More blood was drawn from the patient and sent to separate laboratories for further testing... Western blot, radioimmunoprecipitation, and HTLV-III virus isolation studies were all negative...
>
> Additional testing of this sample on an indirect fluorescent antibody test (ENI) for HTLV-III failed to demonstrate the large cell fluorescent pattern typical for HTLV-III-specific serum but concomitantly identified the presence of antimitochondrial antibodies in the patient's serum. The presence of these antibodies in human serum, as well as antibodies to nuclear antigens, human leukocyte antigen, and human T-cell antigens, has been highly correlated with false reactivity on the ELISAs.[17]

Only repeated testing with more specific tests demonstrated that this woman was not seropositive. The authors concluded with advice particularly relevant to the African situation:

> When patients present with negative clinical histories and positive serologic tests, the possibility of false positive test results should be strongly considered. The need for improved confirmatory tests, as well as access to these tests, is evident.[18]

One of the earliest rebuttals to the view that AIDS was endemic in Africa came from a rather surprising source, South Africa. Blood samples from 139 Kenyans as well as 357 black South Africans and Namibians, 39 white South African homosexuals and 79 sub-human primates (baboons and vervets) were tested for HTLV-III antibodies using the more specific indirect immunofluorescence assay. They published their results in the *New England Journal of Medicine* in May 1985, and in the *South African Medical Journal* the following month:[19,20]

> The only positive subjects were in the group comprising male homosexuals. The majority of these positive subjects had either recently been to the

United States or had had sexual contact with other homosexuals who had visited the United States... our preliminary data show that the agent implicated in causing AIDS, HTLV-III, is not endemic in this part of Africa.[21]

This was followed by a study by West German researchers who published a preliminary report in *The Lancet* in October 1985. Serum collected since 1981 from 3159 healthy Africans and 844 African patients from Senegal, Nigeria, Liberia, Gabon, Zaire, Kenya and South Africa was analysed by ELISA and immunoprecipitation assay. Whilst 28% were positive with the ELISA, only 2 sera (0.05%) from the only patients in the series with clinically diagnosed AIDS were positive with immunoprecipitation. The authors concluded:

...the data suggest that HTLV-III was rare in Africa until recently, and still is rare in much of the continent. It would seem that the epidemic of AIDS in Africa started at about the same time as, or even later than, the epidemic in America and Europe. Our results do not support the hypothesis that HTLV-III virus originated in Africa.[22]

The validity of this research was not challenged, but it was typically ignored by many AIDS "experts" and was never relayed to the non-medical world.

A year later (September 1986) the West Germans published the results of a larger study of the seroepidemiology of human immunodeficiency virus (previously HTLV-III/LAV, now renamed HIV) in Africa. They summarised as follows:

Serum samples from 6015 African subjects without symptoms of the acquired immune deficiency syndrome (AIDS) or contact with the disease were examined for antibodies to the immunodeficiency virus by a combination of an enzyme linked immunosorbent assay and radioimmunoprecipitation (2567 samples) or by immunofluorescence (3448 samples). Serum samples had been collected between 1976 and 1984 in Senegal (n=789), Liberia (935), Ivory Coast (1195), Burkina Faso (299), Nigeria (536), Gabon (1649), Zaire (15), Uganda (164), and Kenya (433). Only four samples contained antibodies. Three of these were from attenders at the Lamberene clinic in Gabon and one from a villager in Senegal. By contrast, two out of six AIDS suspects from Guinea-Bissau, all 13 patients with AIDS from Kinshasa (Zaire), and two out of three of their contacts were seropositive, all these specimens having been collected in 1985.

These data show that fewer than one in 1000 subjects were seropositive for AIDS at the time of sampling before 1985 and do not support the hypothesis of the disease originating in Africa.[23]

The study found that about 10% of serum samples were positive with the ELISA test, but only 0.07% were positive on more specific testing. Expressed in another way, only one of 143 positive ELISA tests was a true positive. Estimates of the incidence of AIDS virus infection in central Africa were exaggerated by a factor of about 150. The authors make an interesting parallel with West Germany:

> In the two collections of serum samples specific antibodies to the human immunodeficiency virus were detected in four (0.07%) of 6015 samples collected between 1976 and 1984 from subjects without symptoms of AIDS or known contact with the disease in nine countries in tropical Africa. This frequency was lower than that found in West German blood donors in November 1984.[24]

The only reply to this paper came from the Belgians, the diehards of the African connection.[25] Confused thinking seems to be their hallmark. They criticised the Germans for including only a few samples from central Africa. Central Africa is a rather vague geographical term, but it hardly excludes Gabon where the largest number of samples were collected, and can include the eastern central countries of Kenya and Uganda. If they meant Zaire, why not say so. They then resurrected the old argument that HIV may have originated in some obscure rural area:

> That most rural areas of sub-Saharan Africa have been free of HIV until recently is not an argument against an African origin of the spread of HIV. Biologically it would make sense if spread had started in a small rural area, which may never be identified. Epidemiological features of HIV·are such that urban life lends itself best to further spread of HIV, most rural areas being infected only afterwards. The sampling available to Dr Wendler and colleagues is not representative enough to answer the question where HIV started to spread, and quite a different picture might have emerged if they had centered their investigations on Central African cities.[26]

Dr Wendler, Professor Hunsmann and colleagues cannot win. HIV, the Belgians argue, arose in a rural area, but serum should have been collected in the cities (where the population, particularly the prostitutes, has frequent contact with foreign visitors). It would seem that only negative blood tests from the entire population of sub-Saharan Africa would convince the Belgians that AIDS did not arise in Africa.

Continuing in this rather confusing vein, they attempted to answer other criticisms of the African connection:

> Other arguments, mainly from Africa, against an African origin of the spread of HIV seem equally invalid. If Africa was the source why was the syndrome first identified in American homosexuals, and not in Africa? An emerging syndrome as polymorphous as HIV disease needs diagnostic facilities, which were present in the US and hardly at all in Africa, and

the early recognition of the US cases was greatly facilitated because they were concentrated in limited groups at risk and not spread over the general population, as is now the case in Africa.[27]

This is rubbish. There is very well documented evidence of a marked increase in opportunistic infections and aggressive Kaposi's sarcoma from a number of long established and well-equipped teaching hospitals in sub-Saharan Africa, after the onset of the American epidemic.[28,29,30] We then come to an extraordinary contradiction. A whole series of researchers, including the authors' fellow Belgians, have established that well-travelled, wealthy Africans are the group most at risk of AIDS,[31,32,33] and in the previous paragraph we read "That most rural areas of sub-Saharan Africa have been free of HIV until recently..." Yet now we are told that the spread of AIDS over the general population (in Africa) prevented it's early recognition! Can these people call themselves scientists?

They proceed to accuse African countries of a "tremendous underdiagnosis and underreporting" of AIDS cases:

> Until 1985 Belgium reported more AIDS cases in Africans, frequently fresh arrivals, than the whole of Africa.[34]

Yet there was a marked decrease in the number of African AIDS cases diagnosed in Belgium in 1984 when specific tests became available.[35] Overdiagnosis by the Belgians would appear to be the real problem. Even "rural Bantu" was resurrected to support their claims:

> The earliest human serum in the world which has been acceptably identified as being truly anti-HIV positive is a sample taken in 1959 in Kinshasa.[36]

This was correctly footnoted as "Evidence of an HTLV-III/LAV-**like** (our emphasis) virus in central Africa, 1959". With such "scientific" methods anything is possible.

Further evidence against an African origin of AIDS came from a group of American researchers who published their findings in a paper titled "Absence of antibodies to the human immunodeficiency virus in sera from Africa prior to 1975" in the *Proceedings of the National Academy of Science*, October 1986:

> Three different assays for detection of antibodies to the human immunodeficiency virus (HIV) were conducted on 677 sera obtained from 1964 to 1975 from male and female children and adults in Uganda and other countries in Africa. Several sera were collected from individuals with Kaposi's sarcoma. No evidence of antibodies to the virus was noted up to 1975. These results strongly suggest that the emergence of HIV in Africa occurred relatively recently. Further studies are required to

determine the geographic origin of the acquired immunodeficiency syndrome virus.[37]

The presence of so many blood samples stored in deep freezers around the world surely refutes the argument that there was no-one competent to diagnose AIDS in Africa until the 1980's. The paper concludes:

> The high incidence of antibodies to HIV was first noted in African sera after 1980. Thus, HIV appears to have emerged in Africa about the same time as in the United States; however, cofactors in Africa could have shortened the incubation period for the disease. This latter possibility could explain the recognition of diseases resembling AIDS 1-2 years earlier in individuals from Zaire than from the United States.[38]

The arguments have now come a full circle. Originally HIV infection was considered widespread amongst Africans who were in some way immune to the infection. Now AIDS is found to be recently introduced to Africans, who may be even more vulnerable than their American counterparts.

One of the original proponents of the African connection, Robert J. Biggar, wrote a review article for *The Lancet* in January 1986 titled "The AIDS Problem in Africa". Unlike many other researchers he has the grace to admit, somewhat grudgingly, that his early research was misleading:

> Knowledge of the genesis of this condition in Africa, its spread between people and between different regions, and the size of the problem has been hampered by lack of data and perhaps misleading preliminary laboratory results.[39]

Biggar refuted a number of arguments for the "Old Disease" hypothesis:

> In my conversations with clinicians practising in tropical Africa during the 1960's and 1970's, they have stated strongly that if AIDS had existed as anything other than rare, sporadic cases, it would have been recognized as a clinical entity. The clinical appearance of AIDS patients now being diagnosed in Africa is striking, and they find it hard to imagine that a condition as florid as oral candidiasis (common in African AIDS patients) would have been consistently overlooked or that its significance with respect to immunosuppression would have been misinterpreted...
>
> Several independent lines of evidence now support the concept that AIDS is new in Africa. Affluent citizens of French-speaking Africa have for many years gone to Europe for evaluation of complicated health problems. Reviews of the records of the Belgian and French hospitals at which African patients are treated show that cases consistent with a diagnosis of AIDS became common only since 1980. Since that time, case recognition has followed an epidemic curve which, on a cumulative

frequency basis, is identical to that of AIDS cases both in the United States and Europe.[40]

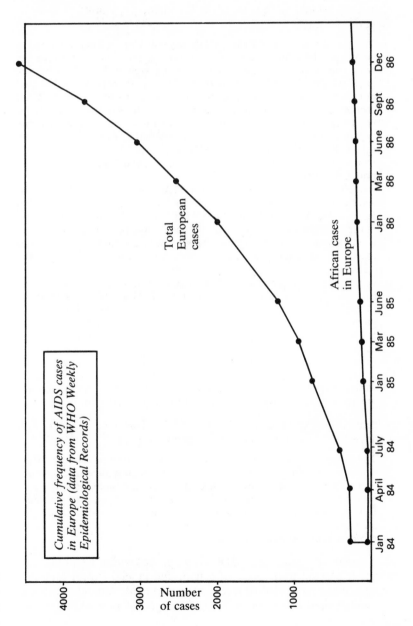

Cumulative frequency of AIDS cases in Europe (data from WHO Weekly Epidemiological Records)

Total European cases

African cases in Europe

Number of cases

4000 3000 2000 1000

Jan 84   April 84   July 84   Jan 85   Mar 85   June 85   Jan 86   Mar 86   June 86   Sept 86   Dec 86

(This last statement is not accurate. The cumulative frequency curves illustrated above show that AIDS is increasing amongst Africans in Europe at about half the rate of the European population as a whole.) Biggar continued:

> The social profile of African AIDS cases in Europe suggests that they were from the affluent stratum of African society. Studies in Africa have been less clear on this point... It might be argued that AIDS has long been endemic in the poorer, perhaps more rural, population that could not seek care in Europe and only recently spread to the more affluent segment of the African population. However, the African population has been very mobile, both socially and geographically, in the past three decades, during which there has been a large influx of rural residents into urban areas. Had HTLV-III and AIDS been endemic in rural areas during this period, the disease would certainly have been observed in the urban population before 1980...
>
> Against the recent appearance of HTLV-III/LAV and AIDS in Africa are the results of several seroepidemiological studies... In studies from Europe and America, 10 to 20% of HTLV-III/LAV positive subjects will develop AIDS within 3 years, and it has always been difficult to explain why populations with such a high background frequency of virus exposure (as measured by antibodies) should have such a low frequency of AIDS.
>
> Recently, the specificity of the HTLV-III reactivity reported in sera from Africa has been questioned. Reactivity may be affected when subjects have had recurrent malaria and other parasitic diseases (perhaps because of auto-antibodies involving antigens in the lymphocyte cell line used to grow the virus) or previous pregnancies (perhaps because of antibodies to DR4 or other HLA types)... Only 2 of 46 healthy Zairean and Kenyan subjects whose ELISA seropositivity was originally considered confirmed because of some form of western blot reactivity had blot profiles regarded as typical of the HTLV-III/LAV profile seen in AIDS-risk seropositive subjects in America and Europe... Thus, surveys in Africa probably greatly overestimated the extent of true positivity among the population.[41]

Although Biggar concludes that the AIDS virus is new in Africa, he believes that it originated in Africa in recent years:

> There is no conclusive evidence that the AIDS virus originated in Africa, since the epidemic seemed to start at approximately the same time as in America and Europe. Nevertheless, it is more plausible for a new agent to have arisen in tropical Africa, from whence it was transmitted to Europe and America, than for it to have emerged elsewhere and spread quickly and widely to involve the general population of Africa and not those of South America or Asia.[42]

The speed with which the AIDS virus spreads within a community is surely irrelevant to its place of origin, and indeed Biggar himself in the preceding paragraphs dismissed the sero-epidemiological evidence for widespread infection of the African population. Only a clear demonstration that African AIDS predated AIDS in America would support an African origin for the virus, yet even the African epidemic (from 1980)[43] would seem to post-date the American epidemic (from 1978).[44] Biggar also argues that AIDS spread from Africa to Europe, yet the overwhelming evidence, including a study in Denmark undertaken by Biggar himself, points to an American source of the European epidemic:[45,46]

> Seropositivity to HTLV-III was significantly associated with travel to the United States in 1980-1 (p<0.007). Travel histories were known for 21 men positive for HTLV-III antibodies. Of them eight (38%) had visited the United States compared with 32 (15%) of 214 seronegative subjects. All seropositive Danish homosexual men visiting the United States had been to New York, San Francisco, or Los Angeles whereas only 16 (50%) of the seronegative visitors had been to these cities. Furthermore, seropositivity correlated significantly with number of sexual partners in the United States (p<0.02, Chi squared test).[47]

It seems that AIDS researchers are unable to remember what they write from one year to the next.

An ironical twist to the AIDS from Africa story was provided by researchers in Venezuela who tested stored blood collected from "aboriginal" Amazonian Indians in 1968/69:

> Serum samples from 224 aboriginal Amazonian Indians were tested for antibodies to HTLV-III/LAV by an indirect immunofluorescence (IF) assay. 9 individuals (4%), 5 of them female, were seropositive by IF and by confirmatory western blotting and radioimmunoprecipitation tests. 3 of the positive sera were collected in 1968. HTLV-III/LAV seropositivity rates varied among the ethnic groups and ranged from 13.3% among the Pemon Indians to 3.3% among the Yanoama tribe. The titres of HTLV-III/LAV antibodies ranged from 1/40 to 1/320. All individuals tested were apparently healthy at the time of study. None of 211 randomly chosen, healthy blood donors from Venezuelan cities had antibodies to HTLV-III/LAV. The prevalence of specific antibodies among Amazonian Indians suggests the HTLV-III/LAV or a closely related cross-reactive virus may be endemic in this area. The findings also indicate that this virus is indigenous in non-negroid Latin American and negroid tropical populations.[48]

The same tests — indirect immunofluorescence, western blot, and radioimmunoprecipitation — were positive in "rural Bantu"[49], and of course this proved that AIDS had originated in Zaire. There was no evidence that these very isolated Amazonian Indians either suffered with AIDS or had transmitted it to the urban populations, and the authors presented the usual explanations of a "non-pathogenic ancestor of the AIDS-related HTLV-III/LAV."[50] Biggar

65

took issue with this explanation, in a letter to the *New England Journal of Medicine:*

> I suspect that the nonspecific reactivity in this setting is most likely due to antilymphocytic, antinuclear, and other autoantibodies, which are known to arise in patients with recurrent malaria... I am concerned that this may be happening among the serologic surveys of retrovirus antibodies in groups living in malarious regions of northern South America and other areas.[51]

This is truly incredible. To find the source of AIDS, a researcher needs only to test blood collected from "primitive tribes" living in any part of the world where malaria is endemic. Surely racism, not science, chose central Africa.

References
1. AC Bayley. *Aggressive Kaposi's sarcoma in Zambia, 1983.* The Lancet, June 16, 1984, p1318-20.
2. ibid AC Bayley.
3. RJ Biggar, M Melbye, L Kestens et al. *Seroepidemiology of HTLV-III antibodies in a remote population of eastern Zaire.* British Medical Journal, March 16, 1985, Vol 290 p808-10.
4. ibid RJ Biggar, M Melbye, L Kestens et al.
5. RJ Biggar, BK Johnson, G Oster et al. *Regional variation in prevalence of antibody against human T-lymphotrophic virus types I and III in Kenya, East Africa.* International Journal of Cancer, 1985, Vol 35 p763-767.
6. ibid RJ Biggar, BK Johnson, G Oster et al
7. WC Saxinger, PH Levine, AG Dean, RC Gallo et al. *Evidence for exposure to HTLV-III in Uganda before 1974.* Science, March 1, 1985, Vol 227 p1036-8.
8. ibid WC Saxinger, PH Levine, AG Dean, RC Gallo et al
9. AJ Nahmias, J Weiss, X Yao, P Kanki, M Essex et al. *Evidence for human infection with an HTLV III/LAV-like virus in Central Africa, 1959.* The Lancet, May 31, 1986, p1279-80.
10. ibid AJ Nahmias, J Weiss, X Yao, P Kanki, M Essex et al.
11. L Kestens, RJ Biggar, M Melbye et al. *Absence of immunosuppression in healthy subjects from eastern Zaire who are positive for HTLV-III antibody.* New England Journal of Medicine, June 6, 1985, Vol 312, no 23, p1517-8.
12. RJ Biggar, M Melbye, P Sarin et al. *ELISA HTLV retrovirus antibody reactivity associated with malaria and immune complexes in healthy Africans.* The Lancet, September 7, 1985, p520-3.
13. ibid RJ Biggar, M Melbye, P Sarin et al.
14. P Van de Perre, P Lapage, P Kestelyn et al. *Acquired immunodeficiency syndrome in Rwanda.* The Lancet, July 14, 1984, p62-5.

15. P Piot, H Taelman, KB Minlangu et al. *Acquired immunodeficiency syndrome in a heterosexual population in Zaire.* The Lancet, July 14, 1984, p65-9.
16. op cit RJ Biggar, M Melbye, P Sarin et al.
17. MS Saag, J Britz. *Asymptomatic blood donor with a false positive HTLV-III Western Blot.* New England Journal of Medicine, Jan 9, 1986, p118.
18. ibid MS Saag, J Britz.
19. SF Lyons, BD Schoub, GM McGillivray et al. *Lack of evidence of HTLV-III endemnicity in Southern Africa.* New England Journal of Medicine, May 9, 1985, Vol 312 No 19 p1257-8.
20. SF Lyons, BD Schoub, GM McGillivray, R Sher. *Sero-epidemiology of HTLV-III antibody in southern Africa.* South African Medical Journal, June 15, 1985, Vol 67 p961-2.
21. op cit SF Lyons, BD Schoub, GM McGillivray et al.
22. G Hunsmann, J Schneider, I Wendler, AF Fleming. *HTLV positivity in Africans.* The Lancet, October 26, 1985, p952-3.
23. I Wendler, J Schneider, B Gras, AF Fleming, G Hunsmann, H Schmitz. *Seroepidemiology of human immunodeficiency virus in Africa.* British Medical Journal, September 27, 1986, Vol 293 p782-5.
24. ibid I Wendler, J Schneider, B Gras, AF Fleming, G Hunsmann, H Schmitz.
25. J Desmyter, I Surmont, P Goubau, J Vandepitte. *Origin of AIDS.* British Medical Journal, November 15, 1986, Vol 293 p1308.
26. ibid J Desmyter, I Surmont, P Goubau, J Vandepitte.
27. ibid J Desmyter, I Surmont, P Goubau, J Vandepitte.
28. op cit AC Bayley.
29. op cit P Van de Perre, P Lapage, P Kestelyn et al.
30. op cit P Piot, H Taelman, KB Minlangu et al.
31. op cit AC Bayley.
32. op cit P Van de Perre, P Lapage, P Kestelyn et al.
33. op cit P Piot, H Taelman, KB Minlangu et al.
34. op cit J Desmyter, I Surmont, P Goubau, J Vandepitte.
35. *Acquired immune deficiency syndrome (AIDS). Report on the situation in Europe as of 31 December 1984.* WHO Weekly Epidemiological Record No 12, March 22, 1985, p85-92.
36. op cit J Desmyter, I Surmont, P Goubau, J Vandepitte.
37. JA Levy, L-Z Pan, E Beth-Giraldo et al. *Absence of antibodies to the human immunodeficiency virus in sera from Africa prior to 1975.* Proceedings of the National Academy of Science, USA, Medical Sciences, October 1986, Vol 83 p7935-7.
38. ibid JA Levy, L-Z Pan. E Beth-Giraldo et al.
39. RJ Biggar. *The AIDS problem in Africa.* The Lancet, Jan 11, 1986, p79-82.
40. ibid RJ Biggar.
41. ibid RJ Biggar.
42. ibid RJ Biggar.
43. ibid RJ Biggar.

44. JW Curran. *AIDS — two years later.* New England Journal of Medicine, 1983, Vol 309, p609-11.
45. M Melbye, RJ Biggar, RC Gallo et al. *Seroepidemiology of HTLV-III antibody in Danish homosexual men: prevalence, transmission, and disease outcome.* British Medical Journal, September 8, 1984, Vol 289 p573-5.
46. J Osborn. *The AIDS epidemic: multidisciplinary trouble.* New England Journal of Medicine, March 20, 1986, Vol 314 No 12, p779-82.
47. op cit M Melbye, RJ Biggar, RC Gallo et al.
48. L Rodriquez, F Sinangil, D Volsky et al. *Antibodies to HTLV-III/LAV among aboriginal Amazonian Indians in Venezuela.* The Lancet, November 16, 1985. p1098-100.
49. op cit AJ Nahmias, J Weiss, X Yao, P Kanki, M Essex et al.
50. op cit L Rodriquez, F Sinangil, D Volsky et al.
51. RJ Biggar. *Possible nonspecific associations between malaria and HTLV-III/LAV.* New England Journal of Medicine, August 14, 1986, Vol 315 No 7, p457-8.

Chapter 7

Robert C. Gallo and some Monkey Business

Of all the AIDS researchers clamouring to prove the African origin of the virus, Robert C. Gallo has been one of the most determined. He is head of the Laboratory of Tumour Cell Biology at the National Cancer Institute in Bethseda, Maryland, USA, and his influence over the direction of AIDS research has been profound. In 1984 he claimed he had isolated the virus responsible for AIDS, and called it Human T-Lymphotropic Virus III (HTLV-III),[1] but this claim has met with considerable controversy and even litigation, and was the subject of a recent television documentary, reported in *The Guardian:*

> All the scientists interviewed in Finders Keepers (World in Action, Granada) were even-tempered and polite but plainly shaken to the core by the behaviour of Dr Robert Gallo, the American researcher.
> He got up and claimed the discovery for his own team when there was already ample evidence that the virus he said they had discovered was the same one that the Pasteur Institute had isolated five months before. The Pasteur team had provided samples of the virus for Gallo — who declined to be interviewed for the programme — but he claimed his own lab had not been able to make it propagate.
> The World in Action inquiry produced strong evidence that laboratory reports had been altered, and microphotographs wrongly labelled, in ways that — deliberately or not — supported the American claim over the French.[2]

With an extraordinary degree of political involvement for a scientific matter, a settlement was reached in the White House between President Reagan and France's Prime Minister Jaques Chirac.[3,4]

According to *New Scientist,* the truth about the claims and counter-claims may never be known:

> The blow by blow story about how the AIDS virus was discovered may never be told. As part of an agreement signed last week between the Pasteur Institute in Paris and the US Department of Health and Human Services, which have disputed each other's claims on the discovery of the AIDS virus, there is now a definitive official history of the discovery. Both parties now "agree to be bound by such scientific history and further agree that they shall not make or publish any statements which would or could be construed as contradicting or compromising the integrity of the said history", according to the terms of the agreement.[5]

Although this highly publicised dispute has cast a shadow on Dr Gallo's scientific integrity, much of his work also seems to be influenced by racial obsessions. Well before the AIDS epidemic, Gallo had been widely acclaimed for his research into another human retrovirus, HTLV-I, which is responsible for certain types of leukaemia.[6] In October 1983 he published a long letter in *The Lancet* titled "Origin of human T-cell leukaemia-lymphoma virus". The article contained a proposal that HTLV-I originated in Africa, subsequently used as a model for the hypothesis that the AIDS virus also came from Africa. It is therefore worthy of some attention:

> HTLV has been isolated from Japanese cases of adult T-cell leukaemia (ATL), some White individuals in the US, and several Black West Indians and South Americans. Serological surveys in Japan have demonstrated that HTLV is primarily endemic to the southwestern islands of Kyushu and Shikoku. Similar studies in the US indicate that healthy carriers of the virus are unusual and chiefly clustered in rural Black populations and possibly native Alaskans. However, the most impressive areas of HTLV infection in the Western Hemisphere are the Caribbean basin and parts of South America... Our more recent studies show that HTLV is prevalent in Africa... In most other areas of the world, and notably in healthy Whites of Western Europe and North America, HTLV infection seems to be very rare, except perhaps in patients with the acquired immunodeficiency syndrome.
>
> ...Miyoshi et al reported the extraordinary finding that HTLV or a very closely related virus is present in Japanese macaques, while Yakamoto et al have found it in African green monkeys... Because of widespread infection of Africans and because of the presence of Old World primates in Africa, we think Black Africans had the greatest opportunity for early infection... HTLV may have been brought to people in Japan by the 16th century Portuguese adventurers and seamen who not only had contact with Africans but also arrived and lived in regions of Japan...[7]

Their theory predictably found support among some Japanese

researchers from the School of Medicine in Nagasaki, who replied in September 1984:

> Thus HTLV of South West Japan was probably directly brought in by the Portuguese or their associated Black Africans.[8]

Gallo reiterated his theory in the December 1986 issue of the Scientific American, backing up his claims with a 16th century Japanese painting depicting Portuguese merchants with an African slave.[9]

Whatever Gallo may know about virology, he is remarkably ignorant of history. Although the Portuguese had limited trade with southern Japan in the 16th century (Japan was closed to all foreigners from 1639 to 1854), they were never able significantly to penetrate this very closed society,[10] unlike Macao on the Chinese coast or Malacca in the Malay peninsula, where descendants of the Portuguese can be found today. A recent search for HTLV antibody in China found only one positive sample from 6884 collected, from a woman married to a Japanese man who was also positive.[11]

The other, and far more obvious aspect of history that Gallo conveniently ignores is the transportation of over 10 million slaves from Africa to the New World over a period of several centuries.[12] If slaves had indeed infected the Portuguese and through them the Japanese, then why did this piece of poetic justice not extend to the more deserving white America where slaves were regularly raped?

Even Gallo concedes some flaws in his hypothesis:

> This hypothesis has recently been challenged by the finding that HTLV-I infection is common among the Ainu people living on Hokkaido, Japan's northernmost major island — an area where the Portuguese did not go. For the time being, however, it remains a plausible explanation of the global pattern of spread.[13]

Plausible, perhaps, to those who wish to abandon logical thought.

As the hypothesis that AIDS was an "old disease of Africa" became increasingly untenable, researchers diverted their attention to the possibility of a monkey origin of the virus. Such ideas cohabit easily with racist notions that Africans are evolutionarily closer to sub-human primates, or with images gleaned from Tarzan movies of Africans living in trees like monkeys. Gallo and his co-workers were among the pioneers of this line of research, both for HTLV-I and HTLV-III (HIV). In the 7th June edition of *Science* several of Gallo's colleagues reported the isolation of a virus similar to HTLV-III in macaque monkeys:

> The isolation of a T-cell tropic retrovirus from three immunodeficient macaques and one macaque with lymphoma is described. The morphology,

growth characteristics, and antigenic properties of this virus indicate that it is related to the causative agent of acquired immune deficiency syndrome in humans (HTLV-III or LAV). This virus is referred to as simian T-lymphotropic virus type III (STLV-III) of macaques...[14]

For those who were arguing an African origin of the AIDS virus, an Asian monkey like the macaque was not a suitable source, but less than six months later the same researchers reported finding the virus in "wild-caught" African green monkeys from Kenya and Ethiopia. This research, like most other research on AIDS in Africa, was motivated only by a desire to prove an African origin of the disease:

> A disproportionate number of AIDS cases has been reported in Central Africa; some of these cases were observed prior to recognition of the disease in the United States or Europe. It has therefore been speculated that HTLV-III and AIDS originated recently in Central Africa.
> We therefore investigated the possibility that primates indigenous to Central Africa are carriers of an infectious virus serologically related to HTLV-III/LAV. In a survey of a variety of African primate species we found a high prevalence of antibodies to STLV-III in healthy African Green monkeys.[15]

This is all very reminiscent of the serological studies of human Africans who, like the monkeys, had a high prevalence of antibodies but were all remarkably healthy. Again, like the human studies, the results in monkeys were greeted with the same uncritical acceptance by the western scientific community. Discussion quickly moved to the question of how the virus crossed the species barrier, and two AIDS "experts" from St Mary's Hospital in London even offered this explanation:

> Monkeys are often hunted for food in Africa. It may be that a hunting accident of some sort, or an accident in preparation for cooking, brought people in contact with infected blood. Once caught, monkeys are often kept in huts for some time before they are eaten. Dead monkeys are sometimes used as toys by African children.[16]

The authors do not tell us where they obtained this remarkable information, but the rapidity with which dead animals putrefy in the tropics alone makes nonsense of these assertions. It is hardly surprising that western AIDS researchers have become persona non grata in many African countries. The American epidemiologist Robert J. Biggar, himself a supporter of the African origin, felt obliged to counter some of these suggestions:

> Even if the virus is assumed to have arisen in Africa, Africans live much less closely with primates of any kind than with cattle, goats, and other domestic animals.[17]

Although Africans have little contact with monkeys, in recent years there has been a marked increase in contact between man and monkeys not in Africa but in the West. An article on Marburg virus disease in 1977 had this to say:

> Monkeys have been very useful animals for scientific research, and with the discovery that their kidneys provide excellent tissue culture cell material for virus isolation, propagation and vaccine production, these unfortunate animals have been caught and transported in hundreds of thousands from their native haunts.[18]

The author described the transmission of the Marburg virus from the African green monkey to man:

> In August-September 1967, employees of a German pharmaceutical firm (Behringverke) in Marburg, and members of the staff of the Paul-Ehrlich Institute, Frankfurt am Maim, and in the Institute of Sera and Vaccines, Belgrade, who handled some particular batches of these imported AGM (African green monkey) and so came in very direct contact with the blood, organs and cell cultures originating from the monkeys, were struck down by a hitherto undescribed communicable disease.[19]

The risks of transmission of animal viruses to humans were also recently highlighted in *The Guardian* by Dr Robert Sharpe, scientific adviser to the British Union for the Abolition of Vivisection.[20] Monkeys, he said, were not only used in medical research laboratories, but their tissues were widely used by industry to produce vaccines, some of which were contaminated with monkey viruses such as SV40, that are injected into millions of healthy people every year. If there is any truth in the hypothesis that the AIDS virus originated in monkeys (and African monkeys are not the only candidates) it would seem more appropriate to investigate modern medical research rather than speculate wildly in such an offensive and ignorant fashion about the customs and behaviour of Africans.

In the January 1987 issue of the *Scientific American,* Gallo attempted to fill in the missing links to his story about the origin of AIDS. Undeterred by an ignorance of history and research data suggesting that the African AIDS epidemic post-dated the American epidemic, we are treated to another "plausible hypothesis".

> Recent results have begun to provide a picture of how the AIDS virus may have come to be... A plausible hypothesis is that STLV-III somehow entered human beings, initiating a series of mutations that yielded the intermediate viruses before terminating in the fierce pathology of HTLV-III.
> That those effects are of recent origin is shown by tests done on stored blood serum from many parts of the world. Tests on sera from the 1960's and 1970's detect no antibodies to HTLV-III anywhere except in a small

region of central Africa, where the earliest signs of infection have been found in serum samples taken in the 1950's. It appears that after remaining localised for some time, the virus began spreading to the rest of central Africa during the early 1970's. Later in that decade it reached Haiti and may have reached Europe and the Americas from there.[21]

We have to remind ourselves that this "plausible hypothesis" was published in 1987. Even the name of the AIDS virus was changed to HIV by July 1986, but Gallo could not apparently bear to abandon his own inappropriate nomenclature. This article was accompanied by a map of Africa with central African countries shaded in "hot" pink to indicate HTLV-III high incidence, and neighbouring countries, including the Republic of South Africa, shaded in pale pink. This is most curious, as the South Africans have not reported a single case of AIDS in a black South African,[22,23] and point to the United States as the source of their problems:

AIDS has been reported in central Africa;... It has therefore been suggested that the agent causing AIDS is endemic in central Africa. However, our preliminary data show that although individuals with antibodies directed against HTLV-III are to be found in South Africa, these positive individuals only come from a high-risk group comprising male homosexuals. The majority of these positive individuals have either recently been to the USA or have had sexual contacts with other homosexuals who have visited that country.[24]

Is the absence of AIDS in Black South Africans the only beneficial result of Apartheid?

Another curious feature of Gallo's map is the absence of AIDS in Angola, Mozambique and Namibia, the former two countries sharing borders with the "high incidence" countries. All three of these war-torn states have had little contact with Americans or Western Europeans since the beginning of the AIDS epidemic, whilst there has been considerably more contact with nationals of the AIDS affected neighbouring states. But then such contradictions are never the forte of the "AIDS from Africa" true believers.

Not only does Dr Gallo seek to convince us of his own "plausible" hypotheses, but he also seems eager to lend his support to other unlikely stories. The May 11 1987 edition of *The Times* carried a story that the AIDS epidemic may have been triggered by the mass vaccination campaign which eradicated smallpox:

The World Health Organisation, which masterminded the 13-year campaign, is studying new scientific evidence suggesting that immunisation with the smallpox vaccine *Vaccinia* awakened the unsuspected, dormant human immuno defence virus infection (HIV)...

Many experts are reluctant to support the theory publicly because they believe it would be interpreted unfairly as criticism of the WHO...

The smallpox vaccine theory would account for the position of each of the seven Central African states which top the league table of most affected countries; why Brazil became the most afflicted Latin American country; and how Haiti became the route for the spread of Aids to the US.

It also provides an explanation of how the infection was spread more evenly between males and females in Africa than in the West and why there is less sign of infection among five to 11-year-olds in Central Africa.

Although no detailed figures are available, WHO information indicated that the Aids league table of Central Africa matches the concentration of vaccinations...

About 14,000 Haitians, on United Nations secondment to Central Africa, were covered in the campaign. They began to return home at a time when Haiti had become a popular playground for San Francisco homosexuals.[25]

At last we learn some details about the elusive Haitians who supposedly brought AIDS to the United States. It is quite unbelievable that the WHO would have seconded 14,000 technocrats from one of the world's poorest countries with major health problems of its own. Whilst the majority of medical scientists were dismissing this latest hypothesis as rubbish, Gallo considered it "interesting and important":

Dr Robert Gallo, who first identified the Aids virus in the US, told *The Times:* "The link between the WHO programme and the epidemic in Africa is an interesting and important hypothesis. I cannot say that it actually happened, but I have been saying for some years that the use of live vaccines such as that used for smallpox can activate a dormant infection such as HIV.[26]

The assistant editor of the *British Medical Journal* was far less impressed:

From the stable that almost brought you *Hitler's Diaries* came a scoop last week that was just as spurious: "Smallpox vaccine 'triggered AIDS virus...'"

The story continued as front page news the next two days, the "intense debate" this revelation had sparked off providing much of the copy. It was up to Tuesday's *Guardian* and *Independent*, however, to record the key words of this debate — bizarre, nonsensical, and preposterous. Dr Jonathan Mann, the director of WHO's special programme on AIDS, pointed out that globally the distribution of smallpox eradication did not fit... The US is experiencing a major epidemic, although smallpox was eradicated there many years ago. As many doses of smallpox vaccine were given in west Africa as in central Africa, yet AIDS is less common in west than central Africa. And there presumably the story rests.

Not quite. AIDS and mass immunisation campaigns have now been linked in the public mind. As the National Blood Transfusion Service has found to its cost, widespread confusion about blood donation, blood transfusion, and AIDS still abounds, although the facts are simple enough. How long will the consequences of this three day wonder be with us?[27]

Unfortunately the "AIDS from Africa" hypothesis has been more than a three day wonder and the consequences are being felt by black people all over the world.

References
1. RC Gallo, SZ Salahuddin, M Popovic et al. *Frequent detection and isolation of cytopathic retroviruses (HTLV-III) from patients with AIDS and at risk for AIDS.* Science, May 4, 1984, Vol 224, p500-2.
2. *The Guardian*, March 10, 1987.
3. *AIDS truce brings history to a halt.* New Scientist, April 9, 1987, p21.
4. *Settlement on AIDS finally reached between US and Pasteur.* Nature, April 9, 1987, Vol 326 p533.
5. op cit New Scientist, April 9, 1987, p21.
6. Scientific American, January 1987, p7.
7. RC Gallo, A Sliski, F Wong-Staal. *Origin of human T-cell leukaemia-lymphoma virus.* The Lancet, October 22, 1983, p962-3.
8. S Hino, K Kinoshita, T Kitamura. *HTLV and the propagation of christianity in Nagasaki.* The Lancet, September 8, 1984, p572-3.
9. RC Gallo. *The first human retrovirus.* Scientific American, December 1986, p78-88.
10. B Moore Jr. *Social origins of dictatorship and democracy.* Peregrine Books, 1977, p228-313.
11. Y Zeng, XY Lang, J Fang, PZ Wang et al. *HTLV antibody in China.* The Lancet, April 7, 1984, p799-800.
12. B Davidson. *Africa in History.* Granada Publishing Limited, 1978, p207.
13. op cit RC Gallo. *The first human retrovirus.*
14. MD Daniel, NL Letvin, PJ Kanki, M Essex et al. *Isolation of T-cell tropic HTLV-III-like retrovirus from Macaques.* Science, June 7, 1985, Vol 228 p1201-4.
15. PJ Kanki, J Alroy, M Essex. *Isolation of T-lymphotropic retrovirus related to HTLV-III/LAV from wild caught African green monkeys.* Science, November 22, 1985, Vol 230, p951-4.
16. J Green, D Miller. *AIDS The story of a disease.* Grafton Books, London, 1986, p66.
17. RJ Biggar. *The AIDS problem in Africa.* The Lancet, Jan 11, 1986, p79-82.
18. EE Vella. *Marburg virus disease.* Hospital Update, January 1977, p35-41.
19. ibid EE Vella.
20. *The Guardian*, April 10, 1987.

21. RC Gallo. *The AIDS virus.* Scientific American, January 1987, p39-48.
22. M Malan. *AIDS in the USA and the RSA — an update.* South African Medical Journal, July 19, 1986, Vol 70, p119.
23. *From the media, Traditional healers and AIDS.* South African Medical Journal, February 7, 1987, Vol 71, pxi-xii.
24. SF Lyons, BD Schoub, GM McGillivray, R Sher. *Sero-epidemiology pf HTLV-III antibody in southern Africa.* South African Medical Journal, June 15, 1985, Vol 67, p961-2.
25. *The Times*, Monday May 11, 1987.
26. ibid *The Times*, Monday May 11, 1987.
27. T Delamonthe. *Medicine and the media.* British Medical Journal, May 23, 1987, Vol 294 p1341.

The Panos Dossier

On 25th November 1986 a new organisation, the Panos Institute, published a dossier called "AIDS and the Third World" which is now being used as standard reference material for journalists writing about AIDS in Africa. *The Guardian, Time Magazine* and the *Reader's Digest* have all published articles based on the dossier, and even some African journals have uncritically relayed its contents. Because of the influence of the dossier, we feel it needs close examination.

The Panos Institute described itself in the following way:

> The Panos Institute is a new non-profit international organisation, founded in May 1986 to provide independent information on Third World development issues. We have offices in London, Paris and Washington DC. We are funded by a number of European governments, the European Commission, and various foundations. This report was financed by the Norwegian Red Cross and the Norwegian development ministry.[1]

On this account the organisation would seem independent only of any significant influence from the Third World. The authors of the dossier were not inhibited by modesty:

> This Panos dossier... has been written, on the best medical advice we could find, for the journalists and non-governmental organisations who inform the public in each country. We have tried to use ordinary language: this is not intended as a scientific text. Our document is often imprecise and incomplete, for better facts and figures are not yet available. It is not comprehensive — but I believe it is the most adequate global review of AIDS yet published.[2]

This is really very mischievous. They claim this "most adequate global review" is not scientific, granting themselves the freedom to make exaggerated and unsubstantiated statements about AIDS in Africa without the inconvenience of referring to their sources. Although they state they have used the best medical advice, even here they feel unable, with a few exceptions, to be specific:

> The contributions made by a very large number of people in both North and South cannot be individually acknowledged here, but are received with gratitude.[3]

The few exceptions include Dr Robin Weiss, Director of the Cancer Research Institute, London, an outspoken advocate of the African connection,[4] but even he is absolved from final responsibility for the report:

> They have commented on drafts of the dossier but did not read the final version before it went to press.[5]

The President of the Panos Institute, Jon Tinker, introduced the dossier in a particularly dramatic fashion:

> HUMANITY'S AIDS FRONTLINE is now in Africa, not in the USA or Europe. This report shows clearly that the great majority of those already marked for death live in the Third World...
>
> In the US, the worst-hit city so far is New York, where one in 250 carry the virus. But in some central African capitals, one person in five is infected. Most of them are in their twenties and thirties, as many women as men, with the better-educated especially affected. These are their nations' breadwinners, the professionals in whom rests so much hope for the future. The impact of their gathering death march will scar Africa for a generation...
>
> And where women are affected, so too are babies. Zambia expects to have to care for 6,000 infants with AIDS in 1987: compare that with under 400 in the US since AIDS first arrived.
>
> By 1991, only five years away, 145,000 Americans will be dying of AIDS. The direct US health costs will be over $8 billion in that year alone, a price which will strain even America's vast resources and humanity. But the health services of Tanzania, Rwanda, Zambia, Haiti, Kenya, Uganda and Zaire must now contemplate today a crisis which is 20 to 50 times worse.[6]

And so on.

The figure of one in five persons infected with the virus is undoubtedly based on unreliable seroepidemiological studies, although of course the Panos Institute does not credit its sources. Yet, without any sense of contradiction, the problem of false positivity of blood tests for AIDS in central Africa is discussed early in the dossier:

> The tests can also give false-positive results: a few people (in Europe about 25 in 100,000) seem to have HIV antibodies without HIV infection... The blood tests carried out in Africa have given more misleading results than tests done in North America and Europe. This is

partly due to the difficulty of performing and interpreting the tests under African conditions.

But even when the tests are carried out in Europe, tests on Africans are often more difficult to interpret than tests on Europeans. This is possibly because most Africans have been exposed to a greater range of diseases; their blood contains antibodies that can "confuse" the test.

For this reason, the results of some blood-testing programmes in Africa, carried out before confirmatory tests began to be routinely used, are suspect.[7]

Rather more than suspect. Wendler *et al* found a false positivity rate approaching 150% ie for every true positive there were 143 false positives. A 10% positivity rate with the ELISA test became a 0.07% positivity rate with more specific tests.[8] We are also presented with the spectre of "difficult African conditions" and disease riddled Africans. The reasons for false positivity have not been definitively established, but the evidence points to endemic malaria, not exposure to "a greater range of diseases", as the culprit.[9] We are then reassured that problems of false positivity have been resolved:

But there is a strong consensus that both the test techniques themselves, and the interpretation of them, have been improving, so blood surveys now have greater reliability than in the past.[10]

We have been unable to find any scientific literature to support this statement, and in any case the authors proceed to use the discredited research to support their claims that Africa is the "AIDS frontline". The only published research using more specific tests has not revealed the high incidence of AIDS claimed in the Panos dossier.[11,12]

In chapter 3 of the dossier "How Does AIDS Spread? And How Far Will It Go?" we are informed, correctly, that the AIDS virus is not very infectious and is not spread by contaminated food.[13] Under the heading "Where did the AIDS virus come from?" we are told:

The theory that AIDS started in Africa, spread to Haiti, and then to the US, seems less probable now than it did two or three years ago.

The first cases of AIDS began to appear at the same time in Africa and the US: in 1981-82. The analysis of old blood samples from central Africa, which suggested that HIV there went back several decades, are now regarded as technically unsound.[14]

In fact AIDS appeared in the United States in about 1978.[15] Extraordinarily, we are then presented with monkey virus story:

The later discovery of a virus (STLV, or Simian T-cell Lymphotrophic virus) which causes an AIDS-like condition in monkeys in central Africa, lends some weight to the hypothesis that HIV "crossed over" from an animal source to man, perhaps when people living in the equatorial forest ate infected monkeys, and that it may have existed in an isolated African tribe for many years.[16]

AIDS, we have been told, cannot be transmitted by contaminated food! It is Asian macaque monkeys, not African green monkeys, which suffer from an AIDS like illness.[17] And where could this "isolated African tribe" be? An official Belgian commission reporting in 1919 reached the conclusion that the population of the Belgian Congo had been 'reduced by half' since the beginning of the European occupation in the 1880's.[18] No doubt many 'African tribes' wished they had been a little more isolated!

Is this really the best that these dedicated 'Third Worldists' at the Panos Institute can produce, in their offices in London, Paris and Washington, funded by European governments and the EEC? Or perhaps this is precisely what their financial backers require from them. The dossier has little time for alternative hypotheses about the origin of HIV:

> It has also been suggested that HIV is a man-made virus, developed in a laboratory, accidently or for germ warfare purposes. There is little, if any, evidence for this.[19]

No evidence, perhaps, because everyone is too busy chasing monkeys around the jungle. It is not surprising that the Panos Institute supports an African origin, as from the outset they aimed to convince the world that AIDS was essentially an African problem.

> The popular Western image of AIDS is that it is a problem for America and Europe. The first major point of our report is that this is emphatically not the case.[20]

Yet the scientific evidence supports the 'popular Western image'.[21] Surely this is a classic case of denying your own problems by attributing them to others.

Chapter 5 of the dossier is titled "Africa: The AIDS Frontline" and contains some sweeping generalisations about the behaviour of African governments:

> African governments have an understandable reluctance to reveal the scale of the problem before being able — and being seen to be able — to do something about it. They have legitimate fears of reducing tourist revenue, of damaging foreign investment, of stimulating fear and racism in donor countries.
>
> The "facts" of HIV in Africa are fragmentary and incomplete. They emerge from roughly five years of unsystematic testing for the presence of the virus. Much of the hard information is held in confidence by European medics, who have promised not to reveal it until one or another African government gives permission...[22]

Let us put the issue of the screening of populations for AIDS antibodies in some kind of perspective. In Britain, like most Western countries, a person's blood cannot be tested for AIDS antibodies without his/her informed consent, unless the test is necessary to diagnose his/her illness. 'Anonymous screening' is illegal, and no seroepidemiological studies have been done, so the real incidence of AIDS antibodies remains guesswork. Blood donors, of course, are screened, but they are not representative of the population, as high risk groups such as homosexuals are excluded. Even patients attending Sexually Transmitted Disease clinics are not tested for AIDS antibodies unless they specifically request it. Compulsory screening is a contentious political issue in the West but considered expert opinion has argued strongly against it, not just on the basis of cost, but because of the serious personal and social consequences that may ensue. Yet the Panos Institute criticises African governments for refusing to publish the results of these 'unsystematic tests' using reagents that are known to give highly exaggerated results.

The only figures any government is required to report are the number of cases with clinical disease. With the exception of Zaire and Rwanda (which are praised by the Panos dossier for their willingness to co-operate with Western researchers) all the seriously affected African states have regularly reported their cases to the World Health Organisation. (Rwanda began reporting to WHO in February 1987) A continental breakdown of AIDS cases appeared in the WHO *Weekly Epidemiological Record* on 21st November 1986.[23] Only 1,069 cases out of a world total of 34,448 (3%) were reported from Africa whilst the Americas (mostly the US) contributed 29,273 cases (84%), and Europe (mostly Western Europe) had 3,694 cases (11%). No wonder those who wish to present Africa as 'The AIDS Frontline' prefer us to consider the results of their dubious seroepidemiology. The image presented of European researchers obligingly keeping their 'hard information' confidential at the request of African governments simply does not ring true. When we have discussed the activities of Western AIDS researchers with representatives of various African governments, we have been told they had difficulty even monitoring their research activities, let alone were able to influence the publication of their results. Many researchers, we were told, simply entered African countries as tourists.

Presumably in an attempt to deflect any criticism from European researchers, the Panos dossier complained about the Americans:

> Once the HIV virus was isolated, and identified as the cause of AIDS, American researchers came to central and east Africa, to search for its

83

origins. By studying 10, 15 or 20 year-old stored blood, they tried to discover if the virus had been present among Africans before the outbreak of AIDS in the US. If it had, then maybe some African populations had an acquired immunity to AIDS, which could be crucial in developing the vaccine.

One survey, for example, seemed to show that 50% of the people in the Turkana region of Kenya were HIV-positive. There were other similar reports.

Later investigation has shown that these very high HIV-positive figures were unreliable... By then the researchers had obtained their blood samples, and departed to do their tests in laboratories back home. They were mainly concerned with the relevance of their findings to the mounting alarm over AIDS in America. Some had no real links with Africa, and seemed unaware of the impact that the publication of their findings would have there.[24]

What paternalistic nonsense. They really seem to be saying that European researchers, presumably because of their colonial ties, understood Africans and behaved in a sensitive and responsible way, whilst the Americans were ignorant, brash outsiders. This is simply ridiculous. When a Haitian origin was in vogue, the Europeans obligingly offered the Americans "evidence" in support of a Haitian origin of AIDS,[25,26] and as this became increasingly untenable, Europeans, well before the virus was isolated, led the bandwagon into Africa in search of a central African source of the virus.[27,28]

The authors of the dossier claim to understand African feelings:

This impact was profound. Articles in medical journals were subsequently re-reported and sensationalised in the American and European press. This jaundiced the relationship between foreign AIDS scientists and their African hosts, dealing a prolonged blow to medical cooperation.

African governments felt that Africa was somehow being accused of starting the worldwide AIDS epidemic. When these results were later shown to be unreliable, they felt victimised... They particularly resented speculation that "abnormal" African sex practices were the reason why AIDS at present mainly affects homosexuals in America, but heterosexuals in Africa.[29]

In reality they are trying to absolve the researchers themselves of racism, by blaming the mass media for sensationalising their reports. As we have seen earlier in the book, non-medical reporters needed to add little to the fantastic speculations of these alleged "scientists". To quote just one example, from the *British Medical Journal*:

To explain how the acquired immune deficiency syndrome can be transmitted to and by women it is claimed that infected sperms from bisexual men are responsible. I suggest that a likely explanation is the practice of coitus during menstruation, which is vehemently condemned in Jewish law but the taboo is often ignored. This may be the reason for the reputed high incidence among some African tribes.[30]

The mass media, if anything, has been more constrained.

The dossier continues in its paternalistic fashion, suggesting that Africans have been oversensitive and have misunderstood the researchers intentions; the "chip on the shoulder" syndrome. Like children throwing tantrums, they have become their own worst enemies:

> As a direct result of these resentments, a number of African states with an AIDS problem refused to allow subsequent researchers to publish their results...(but) information about the African AIDS epidemic continued to leak out, most of it reinforcing the notion of AIDS as an "African" disease.
>
> Those AIDS researchers still working in Africa are now often chary of journalists, often feeling unable to divulge facts or become involved in discussions, even where these could promote a better understanding of AIDS as it affects Africans.[31]

Firstly they criticise "hit-and-run" research that grossly overestimated the AIDS situation in Africa, but then imply that African governments, by attempting to suppress such reports, are trying to hide the truth. And this is all contained in a dossier whose highly sensationalised accounts of AIDS in Africa are based on the very hit-and-run research they claim to criticise. For students of racism, this is classic material.

Towards the end of the dossier, the authors discuss the deficiencies of the World Health Organisation's statistics for the number of AIDS cases worldwide:

> WHO publishes a weekly update of these statistics. However, these figures themselves are extremely flawed. Many governments do not report promptly, or accurately, or at all. The reasons range from the logistic problems of collecting and transmitting such data in some developing countries to deliberate political censorship, based on fears that reporting cases of AIDS will damage tourism, investment and national prestige.
>
> Hopefully, official reporting to WHO will improve. In the meantime, efforts are being made for WHO to draw on and improve the data collected informally by such centers as the US Centers for Disease Control, and the London School of Hygiene and Tropical Medicine. In the present political climate, when many governments are unwilling to report officially to a UN agency, it may be easier for a non-official agency to collect this information.[32]

The Panos Institute obviously fancies itself in this role:

> The information in this Panos dossier, with all its inadequacies, is perhaps the most comprehensive global picture yet made available.[33]

So should African governments, fearful about loss of tourism etc, quietly send off their figures to the Panos Institute? Let us take a closer look at their efforts so far. On page 35 of the dossier there is a map of Africa with AIDS affected countries shaded in. Of 48 African countries, the map indicates that 31 are AIDS affected. At the same time that the Panos dossier was published, the WHO also published a map showing AIDS affected countries.[34]

Only 13 African countries at this time were reporting to the WHO, so inevitably the map was incomplete, but three of these countries, Nigeria, Ethiopia and the Gambia had no cases to report yet all three countries are AIDS affected in the Panos map. Is the Panos Institute accusing these governments of lying to the WHO? Yet another map of AIDS in Africa was published around the same time, by Gallo in the *Scientific American,* January 1987.[35] As we have discussed before, Gallo could hardly be accused of underestimating the African AIDS situation. Yet this map indicates that only 17 countries are affected by AIDS. Unaffected countries include Namibia, Angola, Egypt, Chad, Algeria, Mali and Morocco, all of which are deemed AIDS affected by the Panos dossier. Where, then, did Panos get its information? A few nationals from these countries have developed AIDS, but in Europe and not their country of origin. It would seem that the Panos Institute deems a country AIDS affected if even one of its citizens develops the disease whilst living abroad. By this logic, Britain would be classified as an endemic area for malaria if one of its expatriates contracted malaria whilst residing in Kenya. The WHO is fortunately more cautious. When reporting 111 cases of AIDS in Africans diagnosed in Europe they made the following comment:

> These cases were diagnosed in 7 European countries: 67% were from Zaire and 11% from the Congo. Among the remaining 16 countries, the number of cases diagnosed in Europe ranged from 1 to 3. This distribution cannot be considered as representative of the AIDS situation in Africa since the majority (52%) of these patients were living in Europe before the onset of the first symptoms.[36]

Even when they need to simply copy data from the WHO bulletins, the authors of the Panos dossier are unable or unwilling to be accurate. They state that South Africa reported 32 cases to the WHO. In fact they reported 42, and of course we are not told that most cases were white homosexuals with American contacts, and that none were black South Africans. They report some astonishingly high figures for the rate of seropositivity in Zambia, but give no figures for the actual number of AIDS cases, although Zambia has regularly reported to the WHO. We are then told that Zimbabwe reported 217 cases to the WHO. The Panos Institute claims its dossier is "the most adequate global review of AIDS yet published" yet it was left to ourselves to point out that Zimbabwe had 6 cases of AIDS and Zambia had 217, and Panos had to issue a correction and an apology the day after the Dossier was launched. Even 217 Zambian cases simply does not tally with the very high seropositivity claimed by the dossier, and we wonder if this was a genuine error or a deliberate attempt to conceal the truth.

As we will see in the next chapter, the Panos dossier overwhelmingly succeeded in its purpose. Whatever the bias and factual inaccuracies of the dossier, ever gullible and uncritical journalists relayed the message to the world that AIDS is essentially an African disease.

References
1. Statement by Jon Tinker, president of the Panos Institute, at press conference in London 1700 GMT Tuesday November 25, 1986.
2. Panos Dossier No 1. *AIDS and the Third World*, p1.
3. ibid p2
4. T Richards. *Conference report: The pathology of AIDS*. British Medical Journal, December 7, 1986, Vol 291, p1630-1.
5. op cit Panos Dossier, introduction.
6. ibid Panos Dossier p1.
7. ibid p6.
8. I Wendler, J Schneider, B Gras et al. *Seroepidemiology of human immunodeficiency virus in Africa*. British Medical Journal, September 27, 1986, Vol 293, p782-5.
9. RJ Biggar, M Melbye, PS Sarin et al. *ELISA HTLV retrovirus antibody reactivity associated with malaria and immune complexes in healthy Africans*. The Lancet, September 7, 1985, p520-3.
10. op cit Panos Dossier p6.
11. op cit I Wendler, J Schneider, B Gras et al.
12. SF Lyons, BD Schour, GM McGillivray, R Sher. *Sero-epidemiology of HTLV-III antibody in southern Africa*. South African Medical Journal, June 15, 1985, Vol 67, p961-2.
13. op cit The Panos Dossier, p15.
14. ibid The Panos Dossier, p15.
15. JW Curran. *AIDS — two years later*. New England Journal of Medicine, 1983, Vol 309, p609-11.
16. op cit The Panos Dossier, p15.
17. MD Daniel, NL Letvin, PJ Kanki, M Essex et al. *Isolation of T-cell tropic HTLV-III-like retrovirus from Macaques*. Science, June 7, 1985, Vol 228, p1201-4.
18. B Davidson. *Africa in History*. Granada Publishing Limited, 1978, p265.
19. op cit Panos Dossier, p16.
20. op cit Statement by Jon Tinker, president of the Panos Institute.
21. *Acquired immunodeficiency syndrome (AIDS). Global data.* WHO Weekly Epidemiological Record No 47, November 21, 1986, p261-3.

22. op cit Panos Dossier, p34.
23. op cit WHO Weekly Epidemiological Record No 47.
24. op cit Panos Dossier, p34.
25. E Dourin, C Penalba, M Wolfe et al. *AIDS in a Haitian couple in Paris*. The Lancet, May 7 1983, p1040-1.
26. T Andreani, Y Le Charpentier, J-C Brouet et al. *Acquired immunodeficiency with intestinal cryptosporidiosis: possible transmission by Haitian whole blood*. The Lancet, May 28, 1983, p1187-91.
27. P Piot, H Taelman, KB Minlange et al. *Acquired immunodeficiency syndrome in a heterosexual population in Zaire*. The Lancet, July 14, 1984, p65-9.
28. P Van de Perre, P Lepage, P Kestelyn et al. *Acquired immunodeficiency syndrome in Rwanda*. The Lancet, July 14, 1984, p62-5.
29. op cit Panos Dossier, p35.
30. MH Pappworth. *Causes of AIDS*. British Medical Journal, November 30, 1985, Vol 291, p1580.
31. op cit Panos Dossier, p36.
32. ibid Panos Dossier, p49.
33. ibid Panos Dossier, p50.
34. op cit WHO Weekly Epidemiological Record No 47.
35. RC Gallo. *The AIDS virus*. Scientific American, January 1987, p39-48.
36. *Acquired immune deficiency syndrome (AIDS). Report on the situation in Europe as of 31 December 1984*. WHO Weekly Epidemiological Record No 12, March 22, 1985, p85-92.

Chapter 9

The Response of the Western Media

Exaggeration and distortion of scientific reports by the mass media are common occurrences, but in the case of AIDS from Africa, little embellishment was required. The popular press largely bypassed the 'AIDS from Africa' story, being preoccupied with gay-bashing. These targets were close to hand and thus provided more available human interest grist for their particular media mills. After all only 3 Africans numbered amongst the 731 AIDS cases in the United Kingdom, and all were dead.[1,2]

It was left to the 'serious' press to extend their readers interest beyond national borders to the 'millions dying in Africa'. *The Times* was first off the mark, from October 27th to 29th 1986, with a three part series under the heading "Africa's New Agony". Their reporter, Thomson Prentice, went on safari in Burundi and Zaire and sent back the following report:

> A catastrophic epidemic of Aids is sweeping across Africa, scarring the face of the continent and killing thousands of men, women and children. The horrific picture, only now beginning to emerge, offers harsh truths and inescapable lessons for the rest of the world.
>
> The disease has already infected several millions of Africans from the Atlantic coast to the Indian Ocean, posing colossal public health problems to more than 20 countries. Within the next few years, hundreds of thousands are doomed to die and the inevitable spread of the epidemic out of Africa will add to the fast-increasing worldwide toll...
>
> In the United States, where possibly 1.5 million people are believed to be carrying the virus, 23,000 cases have been diagnosed...

> In Britain, where specialists calculate there are about 30,000 carriers of the virus, the figures seem comparatively puny...
>
> The scale of the African crisis, however, stuns the imagination... For the forseeable future, they will be confronted by a hideous, unmanageable disaster.[3]

The themes are familiar. However bad your own problem, it pales into insignificance when compared with Africa's. Recently, millions were starving, now millions are dying of AIDS. There is no evidence for colossal public health problems in more than 20 countries, of millions of sufferers, but the West seems to have an almost genocidal wish that it were true. For anyone who doubts such claims, we are given the now familiar story that African governments cannot be trusted:

> Individual governments are reluctant to acknowledge the real scale of their Aids epidemics...[4]

And of course the spectre of disease ridden, helpless populations:

> Hospitals are unable to cope with the flood of patients demanding attention for malaria, cholera, tuberculosis, polio and other serious conditions, far less the new, untreatable menace of Aids... The typical African Aids patient, if he or she ever gets as far as a hospital, is likely to be simply sent home to die.[5]

The "typical African AIDS patients" are described arriving at a hospital in Bujumbura, capital of Burundi:

> The patients are gently lifted down from the back of open trucks that have brought them miles along dusty, pot-holed roads. Other people come, propped up by relatives, in battered taxis. Some, who have longer to live, manage to walk.
>
> They are young men and women suddenly made old. Some are babies who will never reach childhood... Haggard mothers with sickly children clinging to their backs pass silent, brooding hours waiting for medical attention. But when their turn comes, there is little the doctors can give any of them but kindness.[6]

On the one hand, typical African AIDS patients have little chance of hospital attention, on the other they seem to be arriving in their multitudes. Mr Prentice's idea of a typical AIDS patient contrasts with the medical reports of AIDS as a disease of the urban elite,[7,8] who are hardly likely to arrive at a public hospital in the back of an open truck.

Remarkably, the next episode of "Africa's New Agony" includes an interview with Burundi's chief medical officer, Dr Cassien Ndikumana. He is quoted as saying:

> Aids is not a very serious problem in Burundi... Tomorrow, yes, it will
> be serious. But today, there are many other problems demanding my
> attention.[9]

If AIDS patients have been arriving at Bujumbura's main hospital
by the truckload, presumably he is incompetent or lying.

Any African protestations about an African origin of the virus are
similarly dismissed:

> Whether or not the disease originated in central Africa — as many
> researchers suspect — or was imported from the US and Europe — as
> Africans prefer to believe — international air travel means that Aids is
> being exported virtually every day to the capital cities of the world.[10]

No credence can be given to an African opinion, and in any case
AIDS can only travel in one direction, Africa to the rest of the world.
But our intrepid reporter cannot confine himself to such generalities:

> (Burundi) is the very heart of central Africa, and at the core of the Aids
> epidemic that stretches right across the continent. Some scientists believe
> that the AIDS virus originated somewhere among these majestic hills and
> lush valleys, mutated perhaps from the African green monkey, possibly
> carried unwittingly for generations among the Hutu peasant farmers or
> the rival Tutsis who now rule Burundi.
>
> Over the past 20 years, as huge stretches of the land were exhausted by
> farming, many thousands of Burundians, among them those who may
> have been symptomlessly carrying the virus, drifted to the capital,
> Bujumbura, in search of work.[11]

There they developed wicked city ways; the men became unfaithful,
the women took to prostitution, two international hotels were built
for travelling businessmen, and the world AIDS epidemic began.
The long-suffering Dr Ndikumana argued that these circumstances
permitted the introduction of the AIDS virus to his country, but such
alternative suggestions were brushed aside. He valiantly suggested
that the difficulties he faced when trying to change sexual habits were
not unique:

> We are trying to tell people not to indulge in *vagabond sexual-* promiscuity
> — and to have just one partner... but this is very difficult here. To change
> people's habits, well, it can't be easy. Could it happen in your country?
> In the United States?[12]

But we are not allowed to contemplate common difficulties in
combatting the AIDS epidemic when African inefficiency and
backwardness are deemed the real villians:

> The Burundi health authorities have had to be convinced themselves by
> European specialists that urgent measures are necessary. Slowly, for

cumbersome bureaucracies cannot be hurried, blood screening is being introduced, and a public health campaign is being prepared.[13]

The British government only recently began its own public health campaign, well after this article was written.

After supposedly discovering the source of AIDS and suitably educating the chief medical officer, Mr Prentice departed Burundi for Kinshasa, Zaire:

Kinshasa, because of the threat of Aids, is now one of the most dangerous cities in which to live. It has the unenviable name of the Aids capital of Africa. Perhaps more than any other city it contains all the nightmares that Aids evokes.[14]

This episode was titled "Nightmare of a Raddled City", a creative use of the English language (raddled means the application of rouge to the cheeks) matched by a similarly creative use of the truth. Although Mr Prentice found the source of AIDS in Burundi, we are informed that:

Some of the earliest traces of Aids anywhere in the world were detected in samples taken recently from the Kinshasa blood bank stocks of 1959.[15]

Are we seriously being told that the situation in Zaire is so desperate that the blood bank is using 25 year old blood! In fact this is our old friend "rural Bantu" whose blood was collected for immunogenetic studies in the United States.[16] Is this reporting stupidity and ignorance, or a deliberate attempt to mislead? Mr Prentice seems unable to confine his fevered fantasies to medical matters, but allows his mind to wander to the racist theme of the excessive, uncontrolled sexuality of black people:

Sexual promiscuity is rife in Kinshasa, as in most central African towns and cities. Many men, if not most, have numerous liasons with different women, including prostitutes... But although public warnings in newspapers and on the radio underline the hazards, few observers expect much lasting change in sexual behaviour.[17]

By whose standards are Africans being judged? Can the numerous 'sex scandals' of recent British governments, for instance, be so easily forgotten?

We are again haunted by the spectre of inadequate African medical facilities:

Medical treatment is fraught with hazards from contaminated blood transfusions, unsterilized equipment, disposable syringes that are used repeatedly instead of being thrown away, chronic shortages of antibiotics, overcrowded wards and untrained paramedical staff.[18]

Certainly the lot of the average Zairean is not a happy one. After suffering perhaps the most exploitative colonial regime in Africa, their very brief experience of popular government was brought to an abrupt end by the intervention of the CIA.[19] Since then the West has supported, both with economic aid and direct military intervention, a government whose capacity for corruption and repression is legendary. President Mobutu is said to have accumulated $8 billion in Swiss bank accounts, along with a villa on Lake Geneva.[20] The relationship between the Zairean government and the West was succintly expressed in *The Economist:*

> If the indefensible President Mobutu is to be defended, his helpers are entitled to impose conditions.[21]

These conditions include the unchecked exploitation by multinational companies of the human and material resources of one of the potentially wealthiest countries in Africa. Little remains for health services for the people. In contrast, post colonial African governments that are a more genuine expression of the popular will have attempted, often under adverse economic circumstances, to reverse the inequalities of the colonial health services and provide a health service for the entire population. Particular emphasis has been placed on health education and preventive medicine, and their achievements have been substantial. But Mr Prentice and most other writers on AIDS in Africa present an overwhelming impression of incompetent bureaucracy whose only hope lies with "expert teams of American, French and Belgian researchers"[22] who, as one researcher admitted to Mr Prentice, have conducted their research for the benefit of their own countries, using Africa as a vast human laboratory where ethical principles can be ignored:

> We must be very careful not just to take away knowledge of Aids in Africa for our own use. Africa has been through that kind of exploitation too many times before. This time we really have to put something back.[23]

On 19th March 1987 *Nature* reported the trial of a highly controversial live AIDS vaccine in Zaire.[24] Addressing a meeting of black health workers in London, a Zimbabwean scientist Davis Gazi made the following comment:

> ...the so-called AIDS vaccine is already in use in Zaire although European and American doctors refused to experiment with it on their own people. But once it proves useful, its availability in Africa will immediately become scarce. "It is not just the use of the vaccine that one has to look into but the way in which it has been reported as well. People have been praised for their bravery for allowing its use on them, but not a single mention of the Africans on whom it has been tested," he said.[25]

Little, it seems, has changed.

Similar stories about AIDS in Africa were reiterated in *Newsweek* (1st December, 1986), *The Guardian* (3rd, 4th and 5th February 1987), *Time Magazine* (16th February, 1987) and the *Reader's Digest* (June 1987). The articles in *The Guardian, Time Magazine* and the *Reader's Digest* were all based on information from the Panos dossier. We will look in further detail at the articles in *The Guardian,* a newspaper with a liberal tradition with regard to African affairs. By this time many black people were angered by the hysteria being whipped up about AIDS in Africa, translated, for example, into proposals to screen students from Uganda, Zambia and Tanzania wishing to enter the United Kingdom. To counter the distorted accounts of western journalists we prepared an article which we sent to Victoria Brittain, editor of *The Guardian's* Third World Review supplement. We were politely informed that someone else had been assigned to do an 'in-depth study' of the subject. To our surprise the prominently featured series contained all the usual racist myths and stereotypes and exaggerated claims of the incidence of AIDS in Africa.

The series, by Peter Murtagh was titled "AIDS in Africa" and yet only two countries, Kenya and Uganda, were examined. In the very first sentence an analogy was made between African humans and animals, with Africans as the hunters and Europeans (wazungu) as the victims:

> The best time to observe the Nairobi hooker is at dusk when the tropical sun dips beneath the Rift Valley and silhouettes the thorn trees against the African skyline. It is then that the hooker preens itself and emerges to stalk its prey: The wazungu.
> The hookers head for the city's hotels, bars and nightclubs where they know they will find herds of wazungu — white men looking for fun and with money to burn.[26]

This can only be a figment of a fevered imagination. Neither thorn trees nor the Rift valley are to be found anywhere near Nairobi (which lies 1,675 metres above sea level), but then a presentation of reality is never the aim of these journalists. Far better to tittilate the imaginations of the readers back home with an exotic scenario full of danger in which the European is inevitably the victim. We are then treated to an account of Peter Murtagh's night out on the town. The relevance of his description of a strip show to the AIDS problem is not exactly clear.

He then indulged in another common practice — ignore the official government figures, and manufacture your own. Kenya had reported 109 cases of AIDS to the WHO [27], but Peter Murtagh claimed there were 250. Such figures, though, are never sufficient to satisfy the appetite of the western journalist:

> However, a more accurate yardstick for measuring the extent of the problem is the number of people who have Aids antibodies in their blood, the HIV positives, as a result of coming into contact with the virus.[28]

Peter Murtagh's "in-depth" study obviously did not include an investigation of the rate of false positivity of these seroepidemiological studies. More cynically perhaps they were conveniently ignored.

We are then told that AIDS had spread along trade routes from its epicentre west and south of Lake Victoria by truck drivers who:

> like nothing better than to round off a day's work by visiting a prostitute. Pumwani, a slum area on the edge of Nairobi, has two flat blocks where some 600 women service their needs...[29]

But then we are told something really quite remarkable:

> In 1980, some of the prostitutes were tested for Aids at their local sexually transmitted disease clinic. At that time, none was HIV positive. Three years later, 53 per cent were and now the figure is believed to be over 80 per cent.[30]

Kenya surely must be the world leader in medical research. AIDS was only recognised in the United States in 1981, and the blood test introduced in 1984. But again, when AIDS in Africa is discussed, the truth becomes irrelevant.

Like virtually all writers on the subject of AIDS in Africa, Peter Murtagh cannot imagine that the virus was introduced into Africa from the West. Yet he then provides information that could explain how this may have occurred:

> When the women of the bars and discos are not hitched to contract workers, there are the European tourists and British soldiers to look after...
>
> According to one expatriate who used to work with Kenya railways: "As soon as word of R&R gets around, the trains are full of women from western Kenya, Uganda and Tanzania all heading for the troops"...
>
> Last year, 600,000 tourists visited the country, most of them from West Germany, Britain, Italy and France...
>
> The port (Mombassa) with its spicy mixture of Africans, Arabs, Indians and Europeans, and the hint of dangerous excitement lurking in every dark corner, provides a temporary home for thousands of visiting merchant seamen and US sailors...[31]

Kenyan prostitutes, like prostitutes the world over, frequently work far from their homes and families where they would face disgrace and social isolation. Any sexually transmitted disease introduced into Kenya's coastal ports and major tourist centres would readily find its way not just to the distant parts of the country, but to the impoverished neighbouring states of Uganda and Tanzania. The other aspect of AIDS transmission that is virtually ignored by all Western researchers and reporters is the possibility of homosexual transmission. We will discuss this further in a later chapter, but suffice to mention here that homosexuality and homosexual prostitution are common in Kenya's coastal ports, and, as in Haiti, there is a high probability that many male prostitutes are impoverished heterosexuals trying to keep body and soul together. These prostitutes provide a direct route for transmission of the AIDS virus into the heterosexual population.

The next sensational instalment of the series was titled "Death is simply a fact of life". Our intrepid reporter had travelled to Uganda to obtain personal accounts of AIDS victims:

> Josephine Nnagingo lives in a mud and wattle farmhouse in the middle of her family's field of banana trees not far from Kyotera, a few miles from the shores of Lake Victoria in southern Uganda... We made our way to Josephine's home as the chorus of happy voices in beautiful harmony wafted gently through the banana trees... Josephine, who is 27, first fell ill about three years ago shortly after the birth of her fifth child... Josephine is not unique in her family. Her sister died of Aids three years ago, as did Josephine's first husband the year before that. He fathered her first two children but her second husband, who fathered the other three, vanished after the birth of their last child. The baby was vomiting and had diarrhoea when it was born but now appears to be all right. Behind the house and beneath a mound of stones is the grave of Josephine's grandfather whom the family believe also died of Aids...seven years ago.[32]

Again the scene is exotic — mud huts, beautiful singing, approaching death, yet the story itself is truly incredible. The accompanying photograph shows a full-faced woman looking considerably younger than 27, although premature ageing is universal feature of AIDS. Her first husband, from whom she presumably contracted AIDS, died only five years previously, but in the ensuing two years she remarried and gave birth to three healthy children before developing symptoms of AIDS three years ago. Even a three year survival without the benefit of expensive treatment unavailable in Uganda is remarkable, but to give birth to three healthy children in two years whilst carrying the AIDS virus is surely a reproductive and medical miracle. And to add a final twist to this incredible story, we are told that people whose traditions include a great respect for the dead have actually buried grandfather in the back garden!

Yet Josephine, it seems, was no *Guardian* scoop. On 16th February, just 12 days after Peter Murtaghs account, *Time Magazine* also published an account of a Josephine in Uganda.[33] According to this account, the 28 year old mother of five, this time called Josephine Najingo, was married to a prosperous trader, one of 50 leading businessmen in Kyotera who had died of AIDS. It is unbelievable that Kyotera, a town so insignificant that is fails to appear on many maps of Uganda, could boast of 50 businessmen of any variety, alive or dead. The photographs were obviously taken at the same place and time as *The Guardian's.*

The Guardian article continued with an account of how Ugandans are seeking the help of "witchdoctors", a term abandoned by all but diehard racists and *Guardian* reporters. Dubious alternative medicine is frequently the last resort of the desperate throughout the world, but stories of animal bones hung at the front door and dog soup somehow make the behaviour of Africans seem different and primitive. Amongst all the nonsense we occasionally find a sensible comment:

> Some people who contract curable tropical diseases are dying because they no longer seek medical help in the belief that they have Aids.[34]

It is little wonder, when flying squads of western AIDS experts, with reporters like Peter Murtagh in their wake, are able to reach only one diagnostic conclusion.

Under the title "Sickening of a Continent", Peter Murtagh

> concludes his three-part study with a plea for help that could become a requiem for Africa.[36]

He described the work of Sister Nellie Carvalho (also featured in the Panos dossier)[37] who has been screening blood for AIDS antibodies in a mission hospital in Kampala after taking a crash course in Britain. We are given the impression that the difficult conditions under which she is working are the best Uganda has to offer:

> By the standards of many hospitals in Africa, the facilities at Sister Nellie's disposal are not too bad. The clinic is solidly built and her four trained technicians are assisted by 13 students.[38]

In fact Uganda boasts one of Africa's oldest universities, Makerere, established at the turn of this century. A chair of microbiology has existed at the Medical School since the mid 1950's, and the current professor is a virologist. Makarere's teaching and research have been highly regarded throughout the world, and it is one of the very few medical schools outside Britain whose qualifications were recognised by the British General Medical Council. Although the University's activities have been disrupted by the Amin coup and the ensuing civil wars, the Medical School and its associated teaching hospital, Mulago

Hospital, have survived as centres for medical training and research. Peter Murtagh's description of the expertise and diagnostic facilities available in Uganda is inaccurate, if not insulting.

Towards the end of his article we come across an old friend, Dr (now Professor) Peter Piot, a leading figure in the AIDS scramble for Africa, who now appears to have mended his ways:

> Dr Peter Piot, who is working with a joint Kenyan-Belgian-Canadian project in Nairobi... says that misunderstandings have been created about the situation in Kenya because the country is more open than many others in Africa.[39]

He is quoted as saying:

> There have been many who came here like the old colonials and drew blood from as many blacks as possible. Then they go home and publish their results.[40]

Such criticisms were obviously lost on Peter Murtagh.

We were encouraged to find we were not the only ones to be offended by these articles. *The Guardian* published a number of critical letters:

> Sir, — Peter Murtagh's three articles (February 4, 5, 6) may not intend to imply by their title, "Aids in Africa" that Aids is endemic over the whole continent, or seek to create an association between this disease, Africans in general, and black people in this country. But I see very little that helps to stop these associations being reinforced.
>
> On Sunday in a Liverpool church, a woman was overheard to say that she had felt uneasy sitting behind a black family because of the risk of Aids.
>
> Can it not be argued that the disease is most prevalent in areas where white domination was, and their black neocolonialist successors are, strongest?
>
> Where is the finger that points to the poverty of Central Africa as engineered by a capitalist, racist, colonial system rather than at the symptoms of widespread prostitution, decadent tourism, lack of knowledge, understanding and facilities? And who is to blame? The old argument of the whore or her client.
>
> Two hundred column inches of, "Look how bad things are; send help," seems to be thinly disguised, "Look what a mess these people have got themselves into."[41]

And another letter, from two women at the Middlesex Polytechnic, London:

> Sir, — We are writing to protest about the reporting in your first "Aids in Africa" feature which characterises black prostitutes as waiting for their "prey". The whole tone of this article, with its gratuitous description of

an act in a Nairobi nightclub, presents white men as victims of a threat entirely posed by black women's unbridled promiscuity.

To homophobia we can now add racism and sexism in our culture's irrational response to this serious disease.[42]

Our own letter to *The Guardian* was not published, but we received a reply from Peter Murtagh himself, dated 12th February:

> I stand over the facts in my own reports in *The Guardian*. The series of articles was not "inaccurate and sensationalised" as you allege. They were based on considerable research prior to going to africa, on what I saw when I was there, plus information obtained from medical experts working there.
>
> Far from trying to "minimise the problems at home by exaggerating the problems abroad," as you claim, this newspaper believes in providing its readers with accurate reports of what is happening in many countries, including in africa.

We replied with a more detailed criticism of the factual content of his articles and a list of references to medical journals which he obviously failed to study during his "considerable research prior to going to Africa". It is always difficult to argue away the facts, and his response was typical of AIDS researchers similarly confronted:

> London, February 23.
>
> Dear Mr Chirimuuta,
> Thank you for your letter to which I do not propose to reply.
>
> Yours sincerely,
> Peter Murtagh.

Perhaps the best reply to Peter Murtagh appeared in 'Letters to the Editor' in *West Africa* magazine. It was titled "Aids in Africa 'a cheap sell'":

> Sir: The very title of Peter Murtagh's three-part series "Aids in Africa" which was recently published in the British *Guardian* newpaper, will have sufficed to prejudice the minds of many of his readers that this frightful disease, hitherto incurable, is an African disease. His first instalment sets a familiar European scene "(suspended flying saucer shaped night club, ballet movements, tights, fishnet stockings and herds of *wazungu* — whitemen)". Using photographic visual aids in the persons of two presumably Kenyan prostitutes, Murtagh sets this scene "against the African skyline" and then proceeds to give the impression that the only source of Aids transmission are the women indigenes of East Africa. How many in far away Africa will read and get the opportunity of refuting such scapegoating insinuations in a British newspaper of the *Guardian*'s standing?

These remarks are not intended to gloss over the urgent need to find the necessary resources for stopping the spread of Aids in Africa and all other places in the world. "Aids", as the advert says, "is not prejudiced". However, in a society where racial prejudice is undeniably endemic and Africa one of its pristine targets, titles like "Aids in Africa" are a cheap sell — "a present" indeed to millions. This could have well-known repercussions. It is already happening for many black people, particularly those of African descent, notwithstanding the fact that there is no Aids epidemic in many parts of Africa.

Just as we seek to protect homosexuals and drug dependents from being unfairly treated as if they brought Aids into the world, so must we ensure that, directly or indirectly, by commission or by omission, we don't blame the deadly disease on one corner of the world. Despite various theories, the fact still remains that there is much uncertainty as to where or from what exactly the Aids virus originated. Murtagh's series omitted to mention this, even in passing, and thus save Africa from becoming the poor scapegoat of Aids. But then, as in many other matters, who will speak for Africa? *Liverpool, UK*

I.S. MENSAH[43]

Our worst fears about the consequences of such racist reporting were confirmed when British fascists distributed a leaflet titled "Conspiracy to destroy our nation through 'AIDS'". They found Peter Murtagh's articles most helpful:

WHILST 'AIDS' INFESTED AFRICANS ARE BROUGHT INTO BRITAIN FROM 'AIDS' INFESTED AFRICA (supposedly to work) TO LIVE ON THE DOLE AND SOCIAL SECURITY ETC (at our expense).... OUR YOUNG HIGHLY FIT BRITISH SOLDIERS ARE TRANSPORTED TO 'AIDS' INFESTED AFRICA (at our expense) TO WORK AS LABOURERS, MAKING ROADS AND BUILDING (at our expense) FOR A SIX WEEK PERIOD. WHILST THERE ARE GIVEN A SIX DAY HOLIDAY AND £200 EXTRA SPENDING MONEY TO BLOW IN THE LOCAL TOWN WHERE THE ONLY PAST TIME IS BROTHELS AND BROTHEL BARS TO WHICH HUNDREDS OF 'AIDS' INFESTED PROSTITUTES HAVE BEEN BROUGHT BY TRAIN AND BUS. THIS EXPENDITURE OF OUR MONEY (and men) IS TO ASSIST THE LOCAL ECONOMY ON WHICH AFRICA DEPENDS... PART OF THE AFRICAN DRAIN ON OUR COUNTRY/PEOPLE. ('Guardian' report.. 3rd February)[44]

Peter Mutagh may not consider his articles racist, but propagandists for fascism have no such difficulty. They do not usually credit their sources, but then how often do they obtain such useful material from respectable liberal institutions like *The Guardian?* The final twist to this story came in an article titled "Highlanders get all clear after Kenya Aids alarm", by none other than Peter Mutagh in *The Guardian,* Wednesday March 25, 1987:

Members of the Queen's Own Highlanders who returned from Kenya last year are believed to have been free of the disease Aids.

...Dr James Dick, health officer responsible for the area where the Highlanders are based... says tests have taken place and the minimum incubation period for signs of the virus to develop has elapsed.

He said: "All the Queen's Own Highlanders have been tested and there have been no positive cases of Aids." ...

A High Commission spokesman said yesterday: "It is unfair to pick on any country and say this is where the disease came from. There was no basis for the allegation that people got Aids from Kenya."[45]

But the harm had already been done, for which Peter Murtagh bears the greatest responsibility. We will now take a closer look at these "AIDS infested" countries.

References

1. *Acquired immunodeficiency syndrome (AIDS), Situation in Europe as of 31 December 1985*. WHO Weekly Epidemiological Record No 17, April 25, 1986, p125-8.
2. *Latest AIDS figures*. Department of Health and Social Security Press Release, March 9, 1987.
3. *The Times*, Monday October 27, 1986.
4. ibid *The Times*.
5. ibid *The Times*.
6. ibid *The Times*.
7. P Piot, H Taelman, KB Minlange et al. *Acquired immunodeficiency syndrome in a heterosexual population in Zaire*. The Lancet, July 14, 1984, p65-9.
8. P Van de Perre, P Lepage, P Kestelyn et al. *Acquired immunodeficiency syndrome in Rwanda*. The Lancet, July 14 1984, p62-5.
9. *The Times*, Tuesday October 28, 1986.
10. ibid, *The Times*.
11. ibid, *The Times*.
12. ibid, *The Times*.
13. ibid, *The Times*.
14. *The Times*, Wednesday October 29, 1986.
15. ibid, *The Times*.
16. AJ Nahmias, J Weiss, X Yao, P Kanki, M Essex et al. *Evidence for human infection with an HTLV III/LAV-like virus in Central Africa, 1959*. The Lancet, May 31, 1986, p1279-80.
17. op cit, *The Times*, Wednesday October 29, 1986.
18. ibid, *The Times*.
19. R Govender. *The martyrdom of Patrice Lumumba*. Neillgo, London 1971, Chapters 17 and 18.
20. *African Times*, Friday May 1, 1987.
21. Editorial, *The Economist*, May 27, 1978, p14.
22. op cit, *The Times*, Wednesday October 29, 1986.

23. ibid, *The Times*.
24. D Zagury, R Leonard, M Fouchard, B Reveil. *Immunization against AIDS in humans*. Nature, March 19, 1987, Vol 326, p249-50.
25. *African Times*, April 10, 1987.
26. *The Guardian*, Tuesday February 3, 1987.
27. *Acquired immunodeficiency syndrome (AIDS). Global data*. WHO Weekly Epidemiological Record No 3, January 16, 1987, p10.
28. op cit *The Guardian*, Tuesday February 3, 1987.
29. ibid *The Guardian*.
30. ibid *The Guardian*.
31. ibid *The Guardian*.
32. *The Guardian*, Wednesday February 4, 1987.
33. *Time Magazine*, February 16, 1987.
34. op cit *The Guardian*, Wednesday February 4, 1987.
35. ibid *The Guardian*.
36. *The Guardian*, Thursday February 5, 1987.
37. The Panos Dossier No 1, November 1986, p43.
38. op cit *The Guardian*, Thursday February 5, 1987.
39. ibid *The Guardian*.
40. ibid *The Guardian*.
41. *The Guardian*, February 11, 1987.
42. ibid *The Guardian*.
43. *West Africa, February 23, 1987*.
44. *Conspiracy to destroy our nation through AIDS*. Anonymous leaflet distributed in London.
45. *The Guardian*, Wednesday March 25, 1987.

Chapter 10

The Aids Situation in Africa

One of the earliest reports of AIDS in African medical literature appeared in the September 1984 edition of the *East African Medical Journal*. A 34 year-old Ugandan journalist was admitted to the Kenyatta National Hospital in Nairobi in August 1983 with weight loss, fever, diarrhoea, skin rash and cough. He was extensively investigated and was found to fulfill the Centers for Disease Control's definition of AIDS. He failed to respond to treatment and died in May 1984. There are a number of interesting features to this case. Like so many of the early European cases of AIDS, this patient also had a history of foreign travel. He had undertaken journalistic training in West Germany from 1965 to 1968, and had lived in London from 1971 to 1979. From 1979, based in Nairobi, he had worked as a free lance journalist for the *Sunday Times,* the *New African Magazine* and the BBC Africa Service, and travelled widely on journalistic missions. The patient's sexual history was a little vague:

> Although the patient had never been married he admitted to having affairs with friends but denied any homosexuality... and denied associating with wayward persons... One interesting observation was the fact that he was regularly visited in the Hospital by his press colleagues the majority of whom were whites based in Paris (and) London.[1]

Given the taboos that exist against homosexuality in most African societies, it is unlikely that a homosexual patient would admit his sexual orientation.

The careful documentation of the history, clinical findings and investigations of this patient contrasts starkly with the sloppy and usually incomplete documentation of African cases by peripatetic European doctors that began to appear about the same time.[2,3] A frequent excuse for these inadequacies was the lack of diagnostic facilities and local expertise in Africa, yet the qualifications of the authors of the article and the immunological tests provided by the division of Immunology at the Department of Pathology give a lie to this suggestion.[4] Whilst Western researchers were "proving" an African origin of the AIDS virus, African perceptions were clearly very different:

> This patient appears to be one of the first known cases of AIDS in the African population... this case is reported to alert medical practitioners to the possiblilty of AIDS occurring in Africans and to emphasise the point that no race may be exempt from this highly lethal syndrome.[5]

Other reports of AIDS patients in Kenya appearing in the local popular press also indicated that Kenyans were contracting AIDS from areas where there was greatest contact with foreigners. According to the *New African,* September 1986, a Nyeri man contracted AIDS in Mombassa, a coastal city with an American naval base and also a popular tourist resort. Another man who contracted AIDS had worked in a senior position at Jomo Kenyatta International Airport in Nairobi. He was described as a healthy batchelor who had "mixed freely with people in Nairobi".[6]

A paper published in the *New England Journal of Medicine* in February 1986 was authored by 12 doctors including two leading AIDS experts, Peter Piot and Thomas Quinn. It purported to prove that AIDS had spread to Kenya from central Africa and not from the West:

> Our results indicate that the epidemic of AIDS virus infection has, unfortunately, spread extensively among urban prostitutes in Nairobi, Kenya. Sexual exposure to men from Central Africa was significantly associated with HTLV-III antibody among prostitutes, suggesting trans-continental spread of the epidemic.[7]

Sixty-four prostitutes from a shanty town in Nairobi, and 26 prostitutes of "higher socioeconomic status" (whatever that means) were studied. The "low socioeconomic status" prostitutes had an average of 963 sexual encounters per year with clients mostly of Kenyan nationality, whilst the other group had an average of 124 encounters a year with "tourists and travelling businessmen from Africa, Europe, and North America, as well as well-to-do Kenyans."[8]

The authors, intent only on proving that AIDS was spreading to Kenya from the central African hinterland, emphasised a significant correlation with contacts with men from Rwanda. Interestingly this significant finding only occurred in the group of higher status prostitutes, and the numbers are very small — 6 of 8 seropositives and 7 of 26 seronegatives. Statistics with such small numbers are notoriously unreliable, and in any case the seropositive group were more promiscuous than the seronegative, although this does not appear to have been considered in the analysis. Researchers from none other than the Centers for Disease Control also questioned these conclusions:

> Kreiss et al. concluded that their data support the hypothesis of transcontinental spread of AIDS from central Africa to Kenya. We believe that the data do not justify this conclusion...[9]

But the authors failed to comment on a negative finding which was quite unusual. Contrary to many other studies, they found no significant association between HTLV-III antibody and the number of sexual encounters per year. Britain's Chief Medical Officer, Sir Donald Acheson, emphasised this point:

> It (AIDS) is not very infectious; you have a one in a hundred chance of catching it from sex with an infected person, but that's one in a hundred each time, so with repeated sex the odds become very high.[10]

The poorer prostitutes had nearly eight times the number of partners of the "high-class" prostitutes and although the rate of seropositivity was higher (66%) amongst the poorer prostitutes than amongst the better-off (31%), this difference is much less than expected, suggesting that different risk factors were operating in the two groups. And indeed, if the information available in the paper is used to calculate the risk of catching AIDS for each sexual act, the better off prostitutes whose clients were North Americans, Europeans and wealthy Africans, have a 16.5 times greater risk of catching AIDS from each sexual encounter than the poorer prostitutes, indicating a marked difference in the rate of HIV infection amongst the clients of the two groups.

Let us remember that Peter Murtagh described how truck drivers were spreading AIDS from central Africa to the coast, infecting prostitutes in Nairobi who "according to research" averaged up to 1,000 partners per year.[11] A close reading of this research shows that the scientists were blaming wealthy Rwandan businessmen (who travel by aeroplane), and their findings, as we have seen, prove very little. Yet this is how dubious science can become translated into public fear and panic.

In response to reports that AIDS was rampaging through Kenya, the British army sought to protect its soldiers. According to *The Guardian:*

> In January the British army banned its troops from visiting Kenya's coastal resorts in case they contracted Aids from prostitutes. Kenyan politicians

and journalists have claimed that Britain is carrying out a smear campaign by suggesting that Aids is rampant in Kenya.

According to Dr Jonathan Mann, head of the World Health Organisation Aids programme, currently in Kenya to discuss Aids control with the Government, the incidence is no higher in Kenya than in much of Europe. So far 286 cases have been confirmed in Kenya and 38 people have died... Dr Mann said that travellers faced no greater risk of contracting Aids in Kenya than anywhere else.[12]

It is interesting to note that only 13% of Kenyans with AIDS have died,[13] whereas in Europe and America the figure is around 50%.[14,15] Are Kenyans somehow able to withstand the virus, or are less deadly diseases perhaps being misdiagnosed as AIDS?

Before leaving Kenya, we feel the issue of AIDS infection in prostitutes should be put in some kind of perspective. The rate of seropositivity amongst prostitutes in the West is also very high, particularly if they are intravenous drug abusers. A West German study found a seropositivity rate amongst unregistered prostitutes, largely drug abusers, of between twenty and fifty percent.[16] In Zurich, Switzerland it was 78%, and in Pordenone, Italy it was 71%.[17] The widespread use of condoms may be protecting the non-drug-abusing prostitute population in the West. A London magazine (published in 1980, well before the AIDS scare) described how prostitutes ensured the general use of condoms in a particular red light district of London:

> He (a transvestite working as a prostitute) abides by the code of practice refined through the informal collective bargaining among women who work the Kings Cross beat. The pay: £10, the conditions: the punter must use a durex. Any operator who underprices or neglects the durex threatens the corporate interest.[18]

The majority of prostitutes in Kenya are economic refugees from neighbouring states (87% in the above study) leading a marginal existence. Unlike their British sisters they are in no position to argue with their clients about the use of condoms, which are in any case expensive and difficult to obtain. Sadly they risk losing their lives.

A paper titled "Progress report on AIDS in Uganda, October 1986" was presented by Dr J. Jagwe, Deputy Director of Medical Services, Uganda, at the Panos Institute seminar on AIDS and the Third World. He reported that AIDS was definitely new, and was first seen in Uganda in 1982/83 and subsequently confirmed by serology and virus isolation in 1984. He discussed some of the difficulties in determining the incidence of the disease:

> Because of various constraints, there were problems of under-diagnosis, over-diagnosis and multiple reporting of cases. Through improved

co-ordination by the National Committee for the Prevention of AIDS, these obstacles have been reduced.[19]

He reported 202 cases of AIDS according to WHO clinical definition confirmed by serology, and another 564 according to WHO clinical definition only, but with no serological tests. He said a total of 250 could have died of AIDS since 1983. This is in sharp contrast to the reports of Western researchers and journalists whose behaviour Dr Jagwe condemns:

> The Ministry of Health has adopted a free and frank policy on the disease. We believe this is the only way for primary prevention. Unfortunately the international media has over-dramatised the situation most irrationally.[20]

Yet Dr Jagwe said that preliminary results of prevalence studies indicate 5-10% seropositivity. In the United States, where the incidence of actual cases of AIDS is 1 per 7,000[21], the estimated rate of seropositivity is 0.04%,[22] yet in Uganda the incidence of AIDS cases is 1 per 16,500,[23] and, as we will discuss later, this could well be an overestimate. Unfortunately Dr Jagwe does not offer an explanation for the high seropositivity figures, but indicates that Uganda is only using the ELISA test. False positivity with this test in central Africa has been clearly established and would therefore seem the most likely explanation for these discrepancies. Wildly inaccurate morbidity and mortality statistics, or a much lower rate of development of AIDS in Ugandans after HIV infection are quite improbable.

Difficulties in reaching a diagnosis of AIDS are apparent in Dr Jagwe's paper. If the WHO clinical criteria (see appendix A) are used, over-diagnosis would appear to be a serious problem. At Malago Hospital, only 15 of 23 patients who fulfilled the WHO criteria were seropositive, ie 35% of cases with AIDS clinically were not confirmed by blood tests, and the real figure may be higher, given the problems of false positivity with the ELISA test. When a group of patients with tuberculosis were studied, approximately 80% fulfilled the WHO criteria for AIDS but only 40% were seropositive. Thus it seems that the WHO criteria, which are considered sensitive (ie few cases are missed), significantly overestimate the incidence of AIDS, and this problem is compounded by the use of a confirmatory test that also has a high rate of false positivity.

The proportion of deaths to the total number of cases in Uganda, at 33%, is considerably lower than the figures for Britain and the United States, which have been consistently around 50%.[24,25] This is an unexpected finding, given the greater facilities for treatment in the West. Unless we believe that Africans are somehow better able to withstand the onslaught of the virus (and there is no evidence for this), over-diagnosis of AIDS due to confusion with less serious diseases would seem the most likely explanation.

Zambia, as we previously mentioned, was one of the first African countries to report a changing pattern of disease that indicated the onset of the AIDS epidemic.[26] An increased incidence of both cryptococcal meningitis and atypical Kaposi's sarcoma was documented in 1983. In November 1986 *The Lancet* published the results of a study of the rate of seropositivity in patients and staff at the University Teaching Hospital(UTH) in Lusaka, Zambia.[27] Sera were tested with a competitive ELISA which the authors say had been shown to give specific reactivity in sera from Africa, although no reference was given to support this statement. An overall seropositivity rate of 17.5% was found, and the rates for healthy blood donors and hospital workers were 18.4% and 19% respectively. These results are, of course, very alarming, and are the basis no doubt of some of the more dramatic predictions in the Panos dossier:

> Zambian doctors fear that the country may have as many as 6,000 babies and infants with AIDS by 1987. (The US, by contrast, has well under 400.) With many of their parents dead or dying, caring for them will be a major task.[28]

Yet Zambia had reported only 217 AIDS cases to the WHO by 30th June 1986[29], and 250 by 13th December 1986.[30] Health services in Zambia are well developed, distant rural areas being served by a flying doctor service. Unless they are engaging in a massive cover-up, impossible in a country as open as Zambia, these figures must be accepted as reliable. On the basis of these figures, the incidence of AIDS in Zambia is less than one third of the United States',[31] and is increasing more slowly than elsewhere in the world, where it is doubling every six to nine months.

The reliablilty of the AIDS tests at the University Teaching Hospital was recently questioned in an article in *New African* (February 1987). The article was titled "Man claims prayer healed AIDS", and began as follows:

> When an AIDS patient in Lusaka, Zambia, disclosed to the church newspaper, National Mirror, that he had been cured of the disease through prayer, little did he realise he was inviting trouble for himself. The authorities at the National Institute of Public Administration (NIPA) immediately suspended him from the college and told him to vacate his room by "sundown" unless he could produce a medical report confirming he was cured of the disease.[32]

The man claimed he had been suffering from AIDS for some time, but recovered after attending two prayer meetings. The article continued:

> His file at the University Teaching Hospital (UTH) confirmed that he had been suffering from the disease, and it also confirmed that in May, 1986, he had a check up which showed he no longer suffered from the disease.[33]

Further blood tests were taken that also gave negative results, but a report from the hospital said he had merely suffered from a severe bout of malaria. The article concluded:

> Whether Chabu... suffered from AIDS or not remains an issue to be settled between him and the medical men. Some people are however sceptical of the AIDS test at the UTH where the majority of those tested have been found with the AIDS virus. "There must be something wrong with the equipment or the people conducting the tests", said a medical worker at the same hospital.[34]

We also have our doubts.

The great majority of Western researchers and reporters on Africa present an image of a continent bereft of reasonable medical facilities, competent doctors or governments capable of dealing with serious public health issues. The only hope for the people of Africa is seen to lie in aid from the West. This perception of Africa and its people, although superficially benevolent, is essentially racist. The measure of the master's magnaminity is also a measure of his power, and attempts at independence and self reliance are discouraged. Zaire, whose corrupt and repressive regime survives only with Western support, is especially commended by the Panos Institute for its co-operation with Western researchers:

> One of the earliest governments to react in terms of research was Zaire. A three-year-old HIV research programme based in Kinshasa is a model of the kind of North-South collaboration which will lead to more effective AIDS control. It is operated by a team of foreign and national medical researchers in close collaboration with ministry of health officials, and with leading US and European HIV research centres. It is called "Project SIDA"... (and) is producing some of the most useful research in Africa, which will help Zaire, and all of Africa, to plan the best response to the AIDS epidemic.[35]

Echoing western researchers complaints about less co-operative African countries, a leading Zairean doctor, Bila Kapita, complained about the "willful silence, refusal to recognise a problem, and misplaced pride among some governments of African countries".[36] This is quite hypocritical, as Zaire, supposedly open about its AIDS problem, does not even report its cases to the WHO, and indeed the only case of AIDS publicly acknowledged by the government was that of a leading opponent of President Mobutu, a former Member of Parliament and a founding member of the outlawed Union for Democracy and Social Progress.[37] One wonders whether the President and not the doctors made the diagnosis.

The results of some of the research that "will help Zaire and all of Africa"[38] were published in *The Lancet* 27th September 1986, ironically the same day that another British journal published the West German research reporting the high rate of false positivity with ELISA and dismissing an African origin.[39] The paper was titled "Natural history of human immunodeficiency virus infection in Zaire" and amongst its 14 authors are a "who's who" of current AIDS research — Jonathan Mann, Joseph McCormick, Thomas Quinn, Peter Piot and James Curran, with a few Zaireans thrown in for good measure. In October 1984, 2,400 employees of Mama Yemo Hospital were enrolled in a survey of HIV infection, and underwent a brief health assessment and physical examination. Blood was tested with ELISA and 152 samples (6%) were positive. From July 1985 the subjects were re-examined for evidence of AIDS or related conditions. Apart from the initial blood test, no other laboratory tests were done, the following reason being given:

> In Africa, laboratory and technical support are not always available to diagnose accurately the opportunistic infections associated with HIV infection.[40]

Kinshasa's major hospital, unlike major teaching centres in the other central African states, is unable to conduct the relatively simple tests for opportunistic infections, yet the whole continent is condemned as backward! (The Department of Pathology at Makarere University in Uganda, for example, was capable of identifying *Pneumocystis carinii* more than 15 years ago at least, personal communication.) Surely all the benefits of north-south co-operation should have included an improvement in Mama Yemo's pathology services.

Without the benefit of laboratory facilities, the researchers used a case definition:

> Therefore, we defined AIDS, ARC (AIDS related complex), and LAD (generalised lymphadenopathy) using major and minor symptoms and signs proposed at the World Health Organisation conference on AIDS in Bangui in October, 1985. Physical signs included cachexia, overall poor clinical health, oral or presumptive oesophageal candidiasis, and extra-inguinal adenopathy. Major symptoms were weight loss (at least 10% of body weight) and fever, diarrhoea, or weakness lasting at least one month. Minor symptoms included persistent cough, pruritic maculopapular dermatitis, chronic headaches, and herpes zoster.

A person classified as an AIDS patient had two or more major symptoms, at least one minor symptom, and at least one physical sign...[41]

This is all rather odd, as the clinical case definition proposed by WHO (see appendix A) makes no mention of such vague symptoms and signs as weakness, chronic headaches and "overall poor clinical health". By these criteria half the world's population could be diagnosed as suffering from AIDS at some stage in their lives. Even the more rigorous WHO criteria are not very specific, as two major signs, weight loss and prolonged fever, and a minor sign, persistent cough, are the classic presenting symptoms of tuberculosis, a disease endemic in Zaire. At least the WHO case definition does state that other causes of immunosupression should be excluded, but such awkward alternatives can, it seems, be ignored in Kinshasa.

In spite of all these inadequacies, the authors believed a valid comparison could be made with studies conducted under very different circumstances in the West. Although such comparisons must be treated with scepticism, only one study showed a rate of progression from seropositivity to clinical disease similar to Mama Yemo's, whilst in three other studies the progression was more rapid. Are we to believe that Zaireans, like Kenyans, Ugandans and Zambians, are somehow better able to withstand infection with the AIDS virus?

The scientific and practical merit of studies such as these is open to question, and whatever the merit, they are valueless if their findings are not translated into programmes that benefit the population. In Zaire the government neither represents the people nor has their interests at heart, and the allocation of a substantial proportion of the national income for health care has never been a priority. The government is, though, willing to allow its resources and people to be exploited by the West to the advantage of Western economies so long as the few wealthy Zaireans receive a proportion of the profits. This extreme form of neocolonialism has been extended to the AIDS researchers, who have been allowed to use the people of Zaire as some vast human laboratory to test, for instance, a highly controversial live AIDS vaccine on healthy Zaireans, inevitably with "the full support of the Zairean Ethics Committee."[42] A strange acknowledgement at the end of the paper we have discussed surely underlines Zairean dependency:

We thank the Department of Public Health, Republic of Zaire, Mama Yemo Hospital, and Ambassador Brandon Grove, Jr, and the US Embassy, Kinshasa, for their cooperation and assistance.[43]

Whilst countries who have raised no barriers to the activities of the AIDS researchers have been praised, the efforts of countries that have taken the initiative themselves have been ignored. Zimbabwe is such an example. According to an article published in the *Financial Gazette* in Harare on 14th March, 1986, Zimbabweans were highly unlikely to catch AIDS from local transfusions:

> Some 98% of Zimbabwe's blood supplies are channelled through the blood transfusion services in Harare, Bulawayo and Gweru, where blood is tested to international standards, including a test for Aids antibodies, according to the medical director of the services, Dr Jean Emmanuel. There are plans afoot to decentralise the blood transfusion services so that all blood used in the country is tested to international standards.
>
> The imported, relatively expensive "enzyme antibody test" to screen for Aids antibodies in blood, has been in use at the country's blood transfusion units since June last year, he said, well ahead of being introduced in Britain and many European countries...
>
> Haemophiliacs in Zimbabwe are not classed in the "high risk" group because, contrary to the American practice, their factor VIII is not pooled but placed in individual packs, said Dr Emmanuel.[44]

Later in the article we learn that Zimbabwe, far from being dependant on outside help, was providing expertise for the international effort to improve the safety of blood products:

> Next month, Dr Emmanuel leaves for Switzerland where he has been asked to be a temporary adviser at the World Health Organisation congress on the safety of blood and blood products.[45]

Zimbabwe is also allocating resources for AIDS research that will have practical, local applications. In the University of Zimbabwe Newsletter of June 1986 we learn that grants had been awarded for research into risk factors for transmission of HTLV III/LAV, and features of AIDS and ARC.[46] The Ministry of Health has a research branch, the Blair Research Laboratory, with an international reputation, in addition to well equipped and staffed diagnostic laboratories attached to several teaching hospitals.[47]

The first cases of AIDS in Zimbabwe were seen in 1985, reported here by the Chief Medical Officer in Harare in his annual report:

> There were no major epidemics. The first diagnosed cases of Acquired Immune Deficiency Syndrome were recorded. This has brought a scare, verging on hysteria, to both the professionals and lay people.[48]

As of 21st January 1987, Zimbabwe had reported 57 AIDS cases to the WHO, a rate of 1 per 145,614 of the population, compared with Britain's 1 per 76,301 and the United State's 1 per 7,040.[49] The

Ministry of Health has responded with an AIDS awareness campaign, reported in Zimbabwe's national daily newspaper, *The Herald:*

> The Aids awareness campaign in Zimbabwe is on with the publication of an information leaflet by the Ministry of Health.
>
> The leaflet, released in Harare yesterday, will be distributed to community leaders from grassroots level so that everyone gets a chance to know about the causes, spread, control and prevention of the deadly disease. Teachers have also been singled out in the strategy which will also involve health personnel.
>
> In simple question and answer form, the pamphlett gives basic details of the disease. It also urges everyone to play their part by speaking to friends and relatives and by keeping informed of latest developments on Aids by enquiring from local doctors and health workers....
>
> To prevent the spread of Aids, the Ministry of Health was testing all donated blood to ensure that blood transfused was free of Aids. Information on Aids would be given through the radio, television and the Press. Health workers had been told to ensure that all needles and syringes used were sterilised.[50]

We are given an overwhelming impression in the West that ordinary Africans are unconcerned about the AIDS epidemic and are unlikely to change their sexual behaviour, that the governments are incapable of effectively monitoring the spread of the disease, are deliberately hiding the facts, and are unwilling to mount a public health campaign. When we look at the evidence of Zimbabwe we find that the government has instituted a series of measures to contain the epidemic at an earlier stage than Britain, and Zimbabwe is by no means an isolated example.

Far from hiding their figures, it is highly likely that some countries are over-reporting their AIDS cases. As of 30th November 1986, Ghana had reported 73 cases to the WHO,[51] yet on 25th October that year, *The Lancet* published a letter from the University of Ghana Medical School about the AIDS situation in Ghana:

> Up to March, 1986, no clinical case of AIDS had been seen in Accra. However from March to September, 1986, an increasing number of seropositive Ghanaians have been seen. 2 presented in March and 21 in September. 44 had AIDS or AIDS-related complex... Strikingly, 63 of the 72 seropositives have been female. Most came home from neighbouring African countries because they were ill, some dying soon after arrival...
>
> In recent years economic hardships have forced many young Ghanaians to go abroad to work as prostitutes, especially in Ivory Coast (a major centre for tourism, our add.) Many of the patients admitted to prostitution as their means of support. It seems that local prostitutes and residents in Accra are as yet largely uninfected with HIV, but that there may now be an influx of infected people.[52]

This letter is reporting 50 AIDS cases amongst 72 seropositives. Unless all seropositives developed AIDS in the space of a few weeks, it would appear that Ghana is reporting all its seropositives as actual cases. On this basis, Britain would have tens of thousands of cases, and the US more than a million.

Although Western researchers may claim that poor diagnostic facilities and deceitful governments are responsible for an underestimation of the number of AIDS cases in African countries, they can hardly apply the same arguments to Africans living in the West. Many of these Africans, for example students and government officials, are only temporary residents with recent contact with their countries of origin, and are also representative of the section of the population, the educated elite, who are apparently suffering the brunt of the epidemic. It is to be remembered that the French and Belgians went to central Africa after diagnosing AIDS in Africans in Europe, because they believed that these Africans had contracted the disease in Africa and not Europe.[53,54] We would expect, therefore, that the pattern of disease amongst Africans in Europe would reflect the situation in their own countries. Is this the case?

The WHO *Weekly Epidemiological Record* (WER), reporting the AIDS situation in Europe, has contained several interesting observations. For example, in the report of 24th April, 1987:

> Of the 4,317 adult cases reported in the European region, 419 (10%) were of non-European origin, mostly African (228 cases) and American (152 cases). A relative decrease in the proportion of cases in Africans diagnosed in Europe was noted: 15% in December 1984, 9% in December 1985 and 5% of adult cases reported to the end of December 1986.[55]

As the graph on page 63 illustrates, the cumulative rate of increase amongst Africans in Europe is less than half that of the European population as a whole, and, as can be seen from the table on page 50, the number of new cases of Africans in Europe reported in 1986 has still not reached the number reported in 1984. In the WER of 22nd March 1985, the Belgians offered a rather peculiar excuse for the sudden drop in the number of Zaireans diagnosed in their country:

> The situation in Belgium is unusual: after being stable in 1981 and 1982, it showed an increase in 1983, followed by a decrease in 1984. This seems to be due to the arrival of many African patients, mainly from Zaire, for treatment in 1983. From 1984, the setting up of facilities for these patients in Zaire, altered the situation: of the 65 cases reported in Belgium in 1984, only 7 originated from that country.[56]

As we mentioned earlier, the Belgians were complaining about poor diagnostic facilities in Zaire as late as 1986. More pertinent to this sudden drop in Zairean cases, perhaps, was the introduction of a number of reliable tests for AIDS antibodies in 1984. Previous overdiagnosis would seem a more plausable explanation.

The French, like the Belgians, were at the forefront of reporting African AIDS cases in Europe, and went so far as to invent some cases in Czechoslovakia. According to the WER of 24th February, 1984, reporting AIDS in France to 1st January 1984:

> Cases of AIDS in Africans patients have been described in other European countries (Belgium, Czechoslovakia, Switzerland, United Kingdom).[57]

The Czechoslovakians themselves only reported their first cases in the WER of 21st February, 1986:

> As of 30 January 1986, 2 cases of AIDS had been diagnosed by repeated ELISA tests and confirmed by immunoblot tests. The first case, a 21-year-old homosexual man from Prague, had frequently travelled abroad. The second case, a 36-year-old man also from Prague, was his sexual partner.[58]

There are many thousands of African students studying in socialist countries, yet at the time of writing not a single African case there has been reported to the WHO.[59] One wonders whether AIDS has a political bias, as only 65 cases have been reported from all socialist countries, including China and Cuba. Ten of these were from Yugoslavia, which has more contact with the West than other socialist countries.[60] A classic example of the irrational response to the AIDS epidemic was recently reported in *The Guardian:*

> The government in the West German state of Bavaria introduced a radical package of anti-Aids measures yesterday including compulsory tests for certain foreigners. All Turks, Yugoslavs, and Eastern Europeans applying for a residence permit will be tested.[61]

The WHO global data to 10th April 1987 included 986 cases from West Germany, but only 12 from Eastern Europe and 17 from Turkey.[62] Either the Bavarians are suffering form a severe bout of xenophobia, or perhaps this is just a crude attempt to deter unwelcome immigrants, who are more likely to catch AIDS in West Germany than their country of origin.

With reports of an AIDS epidemic raging through central Africa we would expect to see a substantial number of AIDS cases amongst Africans in Britain. According to the United Kingdom 1981 census there were 91,586 people from Kenya, Malawi, Tanzania, Uganda and Zambia resident in Greater London. Attempts were made to screen citizens from the latter three countries who wished to enter Britain for AIDS antibodies. Yet if 10% of these people were seropositive, and 15% of these developed AIDS within three years,[63] there would have been nearly 600 AIDS cases from these three countries in Greater London alone since 1983. This is a rough calculation, of course, but no sophisticated juggling of the figures could produce a result approaching the reality — just three African cases, from Uganda, Zambia and Ghana. Details of the Ghanaian case are not available in the literature, and the other two were reported retrospectively in 1984. Britain no longer reports British AIDS cases with an African association which were, in any case, less than 2% of the total. The remarkably low incidence of AIDS amongst Africans in Britain has not, of course, received comment in the medical journals, yet doctors have been advised to place all sub-Saharan Africans in the "high risk" category. The chief medical officer, Sir Donald Acheson, addressed a letter to "all doctors" on 2nd March 1987 titled "HIV infection and tissue and organ donation", the contents of which were later published in the *British Medical Journal*:

> 4. People who have lived in or visited Africa, south of the Sahara at any time since 1977 and have had sex with men or women living there.[64]

Local health authorities also took the initiative. The Bristol and Weston Health Authority issued a circular titled "Collection of blood from inoculation risk patients":

> The following categories of patients are identified for extra care as having an increased likelihood of carrying hepatitus B virus and/or HTLV III virus, and the procedures in this document apply...
> 5. Patients who have visited Zaire, Zambia, Uganda in the last 5 years.[65]

Dr Pinching, a particularly vociferous supporter of the African origin, made the following recommendation for obstetrics patients:

> Women should also be screened if they or their sexual partners have recently resided in Central Africa, where the disease is thought to have originated and where the infection rate is high. These countries include Zaire, Zambia, Uganda and Rwanda.[66]

Surely Dr Pinching would have expected to see at least a few score of African patients at St Mary's Hospital in London, from where he makes such confident pronouncements. As a member of the Department of Health and Social Security's advisory committee on AIDS, he is in a position to influence the government's stance on AIDS in Africa. His colleague at St Mary's, virologist Dr D J Jeffries is rather more cautious. He made the following comment about an AIDS educational video that claimed the virus originated in Africa:

While the good points far outweigh its disadvantages, the film has one or two weaknesses. Many people are curious as to the origin of the virus, but without further evidence it seems unfair to perpetuate the suggestion that the virus was taken by Haitian migrants from Zaire to Haiti.[67]

Dr Pinching's racial obsessions received a further airing in *The Lancet*, May 1987. He claimed to have discovered a genetic variant that predisposed the person to infection with the AIDS virus. He further claimed that this particular gene type was common in central Africa:

It is of interest that in an area where HIV infection is very common — namely, in some parts of Central Africa — the Gc 1f allele predominates in the indigenous population (table IV).[68]

Table IV, we discover, was footnoted in the following way:

From Constans J, et al, personal communication; subjects included Caucasians from France, Germany and Switzerland... No geographic information on subjects (from Central Africa) available.[69]

Support for a hypothesis that Africans have a racial predisposition to AIDS is provided by unpublished data collected from unknown Africans from unknown locations for unknown reasons. This piece of "research" was reported in the media as a major breakthrough in the search for a cure for AIDS.

One of the most respected AIDS scientists, Professor Michael Adler, urged caution over the interpretation of Dr Pinching's research:

There may be genetically determined differences in susceptibility to infection that affect transmission risks between subjects and within populations of different ethnic origin. Such hypotheses can be tested only by further careful research.

The medical profession must be honest about its own current areas of ignorance, but the media watching public must also be prepared to accept the uncertainties of the questions scientific endeavour has yet to answer.[70]

How much better for Africa if all the scientists studying AIDS followed this sound advice.

References
1.   AOK Obel, SK Sharif, SO McLigeyo et al. *Acquired immunodeficiency syndrome in an African.* East African Medical Journal, September 1984, Vol 61 No 9, p724-6.
2.   P Piot, H Taelman, KB Minlange et al. *Acquired immunodeficiency syndrome in a heterosexual population in Zaire.* The Lancet, July 14, 1984, p65-9.

3. P Van de Perre, P Lepage, P Kestelyn et al. *Acquired immunodeficiency syndrome in Rwanda.* The Lancet, July 14, 1984, p62-5.
4. P Harrison. *Inside the Third World.* Penguin Books Ltd, 1979, p281-302
5. op cit AOK Obel, SK Sharif, SO McLigeyo et al.
6. *Kenya shudders from AIDS fright.* New African, September 1986, p31.
7. JK Kreiss, D Koech, P Piot, TC Quinn et al. *AIDS virus infection in Nairobi prostitutes. Spread of the epidemic to East Africa.* New England Journal of Medicine, February 13, 1986, Vol 314 No 7, p414-8.
8. ibid JK Kreiss, D Koech, P Piot, TC Quinn et al.
9. DN Forthal, A Friede. *HTLV-III antibody in east Africa.* New England Journal of Medicine, July 24, 1986, Vol 315 No 4, p259.
10. Quoted in *The Guardian,* Monday March 9, 1987.
11. *The Guardian*, Tuesday February 3, 1987.
12. *The Guardian*, Thursday March 12, 1987.
13. *The Guardian*, Thursday March 12, 1987.
14. *Acquired immunodeficiency syndrome (AIDS) — update. (United States of America).* WHO Weekly Epidemiological Record No 6, February 6, 1987, p29-36.
15. *Situation in the WHO European region as of 31 December 1986.* WHO Weekly Epidemiological Record No 17, April 24, 1987, p117-24.
16. WA Haseltine. *HTLV-III/LAV-antibody-positive soldiers in Berlin.* New England Journal of Medicine, Jan 2, 1986, Vol 314 No 1, p55-6.
17. Centers for Disease Control. *Antibody to Human Immunodeficiency Virus in Female Prostitutes.* Morbidity and Mortality Weekly Report, March 27, 1987, Vol 36, No 11, p157-61.
18. *One way ticket.* Time Out, May 30 — June 6, 1980.
19. JGM Jagwe. *Progress report on AIDS in Uganda, October 1986.* The Panos Institute, London.
20. ibid JGM Jagwe.
21. These figures were calculated from the WHO Weekly Epidemiological Record No 15, April 10, 1987. *Acquired immunodeficiency syndrome (AIDS) Global Data*, and Whitaker's Almanack 1987, The Year Book, 119th edition, London.
22. DM Barnes. *Military statistics on AIDS in the U.S.* Science, July 18, 1986, Vol 233 p283.
23. op cit WHO Weekly Epidemiological Record No 15, April 10, 1987, and Whitaker's Almanack 1987, The Year Book, 119th edition, London.
24. op cit WHO Weekly Epidemiological Record No 6, February 6, 1987.
25. op cit WHO Weekly Epidemiological Record No 17, April 24, 1987
26. AC Bayley. *Aggressive Kaposi's sarcoma in Zambia, 1983.* The Lancet, June 16, 1984, p1318-20.
27. M Melbye, A Bayley, RA Weiss, RJ Biggar et al. *Evidence for heterosexual transmission and clinical manifestations of human immunodeficiency virus infection and related conditions in Lusaka, Zambia.* The Lancet, November 15, 1986, p1113-5.
28. The Panos Dossier, p38.
29. *Acquired immunodeficiency syndrome (AIDS) Global data,* WHO Weekly Epidemiological Record No 47, November 21, 1986, p361-8.

30. *Acquired immunodeficiency syndrome (AIDS) Global data.* WHO Weekly Epidemiological Record No 3, January 16, 1987, p10.
31. op cit WHO Weekly Epidemiological Record No 15, April 10, 1987, and Whitaker's Almanack 1987, The Year Book, 119th edition, London.
32. *Man claims prayer healed AIDS.* New African, February 1987.
33. ibid *Man claims prayer healed AIDS.*
34. ibid *Man claims prayer healed AIDS.*
35. The Panos Dossier, p41.
36. DM Barnes. *Unsuspected prevalence of AIDS in Africa.* Science, July 18, 1986, Vol 233 p282.
37. *Zairean opposition leader dies.* African Times, Friday March 27, 1987.
38. op cit The Panos Dossier, p41.
39. I Wendler, J Schneider, B Gras et al. *Seroepidemiology of human immunodeficiency virus in Africa.* British Medical Journal, September 27, 1986, Vol 293 p782-5.
40. JM Mann, RL Colebunders, TC Quinn, P Piot, JW Curran et al. *Natural history of human immunodeficiency virus in Zaire.* The Lancet, September 27, 1986, p707-9.
41. ibid JM Mann, RL Colebunders, TC Quinn, P Piot, JW Curran et al.
42. D Zagury, R Leonard, M Fouchard, B Reveil. *Immunisation against AIDS in humans.* Nature, March 19, 1987, Vol 326 p249-50.
43. ibid JM Mann, RL Colebunders, TC Quinn, P Piot, JW Curran et al.
44. *Virtually no risk of Aids from local transfusions, says expert.* Financial Gazette, Harare, March 14, 1986.
45. ibid Financial Gazette, Harare, March 14, 1986.
46. University of Zimbabwe Newsletter, No 37, June 1986, p30.
47. J Gilmurray, R Riddell, D Sanders. *From Rhodesia to Zimbabwe No 7 "The struggle for health".* Catholic Institute for International Relations, London, 1979.
48. *Report of the City Health Department: 1985.* City Health Department, Harare, April 15, 1986.
49. op cit WHO Weekly Epidemiological Record No 15, April 10, 1987, and Whitaker's Almanack 1987, The Year Book, 119th edition, London.
50. *Ministry of Health launches pamphlets on Aids awareness.* The Herald, Harare, Tuesday March 31, 1987.
51. op cit *Acquired immunodeficiency syndrome (AIDS) Global data.* WHO Weekly Epidemiological Record No 3, January 16, 1987.
52. AR Neequaye, J Neequaye, JA Mingle, D Ofori Adjei. *Preponderance of females with AIDS in Ghana.* The Lancet, October 25, 1986, p978.
53. op cit P Piot, H Taelman, KB Minlange et al.
54. op cit P Van de Perre, P Lepage, P Kestelyn et al.
55. op cit WHO Weekly Epidemiological Record No 17, April 24, 1987.
56. *Acquired immunodeficiency syndrome (AIDS). Report on the situation in Europe as of 31 December 1984.* WHO Weekly Epidemiological Record No 12, March 22, 1985, p85-90.
57. *Acquired immune deficiency syndrome (AIDS) France.* WHO Weekly Epidemiological Record No 8, February 24, 1984, p57-8.
58. *Acquired immune deficiency syndrome (AIDS), Czechoslovakia.* WHO

Weekly Epidemiological Record No 8, February 21, 1986, p59.

59. *Acquired immunodeficiency syndrome (AIDS) Global Data.* WHO Weekly Epidemiological Record No 15, April 10, 1987, p101-3.
60. op cit WHO Weekly Epidemiological Record No 15, April 10, 1987.
61. *The Guardian*, May 20, 1987.
62. op cit WHO Weekly Epidemiological Record No 15, April 10, 1987.
63. RJ Biggar. *The AIDS problem in Africa.* The Lancet, January 11, 1986, p79-82. (Biggar states that 10-20% of seropositive subjects will develop AIDS within 3 years).
64. AM Johnson, MW Adler. *ABC of AIDS, Strategies for prevention.* British Medical Journal, August 8, Vol 295 p373-6.
65. Bristol and Weston Health Authority medical staff information sheet, Vol 3 No 9, September 1985, p21.
66. H Cudby. *The AIDS virus, obstetrics and the newborn.* The British Journal for Nurses in Child Health, June 1986, Vol 1 No 4, p112-3.
67. DJ Jeffries. *Medicine and the media.* British Medical Journal, October 11, 1986, Vol 293 p951.
68. L-J Eales, JM Parkin, AJ Pinching et al. *Association of different allelic forms of group specific component with susceptibility to and clinical manifestation of human immunodeficiency virus infection.* The Lancet, May 2 1987, p999-1002.
69. ibid L-J Eales, JM Parkin, AJ Pinching et al.
70. AM Johnson, MW Adler. *AIDS and the heterosexual epidemic.* British Medical Journal, May 23, 1987, Vol 294 p1354.

Chapter 11

The African Media Replies

Many Africans responded vigorously to the suggestion that they were responsible for infecting the world with AIDS, but predictably their voices were ignored in the West. Well researched articles appeared in a number of African newspapers and magazines, and African scientists and government officials voiced their protests at international scientific meetings on AIDS. An international conference held in Dakar, Senegal, in 1985 provided a platform for some of the most persistent proponents of the African connection, and was the subject of a report by Yinka Adeyemi, the science and health correspondent for the Nigerian weekly, *Concord*. He began:

> To the average European researcher in virus cancers, the notion that the Acquired Immune Deficiency Syndrome (AIDS) had its origin in Africa is now a scientific fact... Yet, arguments by such scientists whose minds are made up about the African connection are replete with fundamental loopholes and illogicalities that render them not plausible.[1]

He was well acquainted with the current scientific literature on the subject, and was highly critical, particularly of Dr Kevin De Cock and the Belgian researchers in Zaire and Rwanda:

> It is argued for instance that the 'African connection' school is guilty of selection bias. Critics ask: What prompted the researchers to go to Zaire and Kigali and not New York, San Francisco and many Scandinavian cities — where the outbreak of AIDS is equally alarming? (He is referring to the situation in Denmark, our add).
> Besides, says Wemimo Benson of the Lagos University Teaching Hospital, it amounts to saying nothing if researchers went to cities where a disease is generally believed to be endemic, and based on certain symptoms, conclude that such a disease is rampant in those cities.

Critics also say that it is very likely that scientists who subscribe to the "African connection" theory may have inadvertently mistaken AIDS symptoms for other diseases exhibiting similar symptoms... malaria fever, pneumonia and tuberculosis.[2]

He commented on the racist underpinnings of Western research:

A common notion which cuts through the reasoning of most Western scientists is that a visit should be made to Africa before any researcher concludes whether a disease is new. For instance, De Cock wrote that Ebola virus, Marburg virus and lassa fever were all initially thought to be new diseases when they first surfaced "but all of them turned out to have been endemic in Africa."

There are even more offensive notions... Gallo, who first identified the AIDS-causing virus in man, said at the Dakar conference: "Viruses closely related to HTLV, but distinct from it, have been isolated from Old World monkeys. This and other facts led us to propose that the ancestral origin of HTLV is in Africa."

Comments such as this immediately raise problems because of the socio-historical implications. To the ordinary man, Gallo will be understood as saying that: "We (European scientists) conclude that AIDS originated from Africa because we found AIDS virus in monkeys, and Africans are closer to monkeys."[3]

He argued that African scientists should counteract Western AIDS research, and felt they had been insufficiently critical:

The task of such research falls on African scientists and particularly the Scientific and Technical Commission of the Organisation of African Unity... Unfortunately (few) have dared to challenge the conclusions of European scientists with respect to the origin of AIDS.[4]

By November 1985, the situation had changed. A symposium on AIDS held in Brussels was reported in the January 1986 edition of *New African:*

By the close of the two-day symposium on AIDS in Africa held in Brussels, a stand-off had developed between some Western medical scientists who insisted that the disease was spreading through Africa and, indeed, might well have begun there, and African scientists and government officials who maintained it was unproductive to stress the disease's 'African connection'.[5]

The meeting was apparently so fractious that the African representatives felt obliged to issue their own statement:

The 50 African representatives from 15 African countries issued a communique at the end of the meeting which stated: 'The symposium did not show any conclusive evidence that AIDS originated in Africa. Therefore, efforts directed at associating Africa with AIDS do not contribute to future control programmes.'

The African representatives also dismissed what many scientists take to be an important link between AIDS in Central Africa and the occurrence of Kaposi's sarcoma, a form of skin cancer. Kaposi's sarcoma has long been endemic to Central Africa, but has occurred rarely in Europe and the USA until it began afflicting a high proportion of AIDS sufferers. However, the Africans' communique in Brussels denied that any relationship had been proved between AIDS and Kaposi's sarcoma.

The communique went on to point out that the test for presence of the AIDS virus used in Africa is unreliable and gives a falsely high number of positive results. The document also said that so far, all evidence that the disease originated in a virus common to Green Monkeys was merely hypothetical, and that there are other, equally tenable, hypotheses concerning the disease's origins.[6]

African scientists also rejected accusations of complacency:

> But despite their opposition to Western scientist's theories linking Africa with the origin of AIDS, the African representatives did not take a 'head in the sand' attitude, as some of their critics accused. In their communique, the African group called for help to install safe blood-banks to minimalise the risk of AIDS being transmitted through blood transfusions. They also called for help in setting up cheap laboratory methods to diagnose the disease.[7]

In stark contrast to the reporting of African AIDS in the Western press, this issue of *New African* presented detailed and accurate information about the AIDS situation:

> Across a swathe of Central Africa is an area known as the Lymphoma belt, so named because of the high prevalence of lymph disorders in the region, with Burkitt's lymphoma and Kaposi's sarcoma amongst the most common. Although it accounts for a sixth of all malignancies in some parts of this area, Kaposi's sarcoma is generally an indolent disease, often affecting only the hands and feet, proving responsive to drug treatment and rarely proving fatal. In Western AIDS cases, however, Kaposi's sarcoma spreads rapidly and aggressively throughout the whole body and, as with other infections which attack the body whose defences have been destroyed by the AIDS virus, it is not responsive to treatment...
>
> Even the procedures used in diagnostic testing for the presence of the AIDS virus in the blood — which were developed in the West, largely for Western patients — are now suspected of giving false positive results when African serum is tested. This is particularly the case in regions where malaria is endemic. This is because people living in such regions tend to develop high concentrations of malaria antibodies in their blood which may be cross-reacting with the AIDS test, thus giving erroneous results...
>
> Testing blood serum which has been frozen for storage has proved particularly problematic, and claims that the AIDS virus has been identified in sera which dates back to the 1950's need to be studied very closely.[8]

Western governments were obviously listening to arguments very different from those presented in the African media, and when proposals were made to screen Africans seeking entry into European countries, the response was angry. The editorial of the 2nd April issue of *The Herald* in Zimbabwe contained the following comments:

There is every indication that the Aids scourge could leave this world dangerously polarised between the white North and the black South.

That is how any intelligent person will interpret the ethno-centricism and open racism which are rearing their ugly heads in the wake of the Aids syndrome.

First, futile attempts, backed by dubious scientific claims, were made by the West to pinpoint Africa as the place where Aids originated. Then some countries in the Northern hemisphere tried to impose restrictions on visitors from some African countries unless these people were first certified free from Aids in their own countries.

Now there are even more disturbing reports to the effect that some European countries will not allow African students entry to take up scholarships unless the students produce certificates in advance giving them a clean bill of health.

If these moves are genuinely intended to check the spread of Aids, one wonders why students from other European countries where Aids is also known to be as prevalent as it is in some African states, are not affected by the same restrictions? Or why the United States of America, where the highest number of Aids cases has been reported, has not found it necessary to curb visits by Africans there?

The trend in Europe is hideous and worrying. If allowed to continue, it could lead to most, if not all, European countries getting rid of African students by using Aids as a scapegoat, and with that the aid these countries give to Africa. Other countries whose ethnocentric or racist views are known to all, might also use the Aids pretext to clamp down on immigrants.

In the light of all this, it will not surprise anyone if some African countries are found to withhold information on Aids for fear of repercussions from European countries on whom some depend helplessly for financial and other assistance.

What is needed is not to divide the world, but to foster the closest co-operation in battling humankind's common enemy, Aids.[9]

A leading Kenyan columnist, Philip Ochieng, made similar, but more detailed comments in the January 1987 issue of *New African:*

The British Government's threat to subject visitors from certain African countries to "screening" against AIDS is remarkable in its disregard for the consequences. There was a time when Britain could propose such a blatantly discriminatory programme and get away with it — but that time has long past...

What is suggested in Britain's latest move is that these countries have not only the biggest number of AIDS cases in the world but that the disease itself originated from here...

Why is it that we had never heard of AIDS or anything approaching it until after it appeared in the US and Europe? Why is it that those areas of Africa most in contact with Europeans and Americans over the past 15 years are the worst affected by AIDS? What is the only logical conclusion to draw?

Again the methods used to determine the spread of AIDS in the West and in Africa are vastly different. In the West the emphasis is on actual cases reported and projections based on lifestyles. In Africa, a few people, mostly prostitutes, are rounded up and subjected to screening. Whenever AIDS *antibodies* are discovered, the medical boffins juggle their calculators and come up with figures that suggest that half the entire nation is suffering from AIDS! If the same system of calculation was applied to California, the results might well indicate that every citizen there had not only contracted AIDS but had died from it!

It seems to me that the West was once again looking for a whipping boy when AIDS first emerged and Africa, as usual, was convenient.

Unfortunately for the West, this line will no longer wash in Africa. In fact Africa and other Third World countries should think twice before allowing Americans and Europeans past their borders. If Britain is really concerned about the spread of AIDS, then it should screen its own citizens before allowing them to depart to other countries lest they carry their deadly virus with them...

To single out Central African countries as potential AIDS carriers on the flimsiest of evidence is nothing but racism. It is only another attempt to bar the entry of coloured immigrants into Britain. It comes in the wake of visa impositions on the black Commonwealth countries...[11]

In conclusion, he warns against the consequences of such attempts at screening:

Any selective war on AIDS especially when it is couched in terms which smack of racism can only anger other parts of the world, making co-operation impossible, and thus enhancing the survival chances of this new and deadly virus.[11]

If any Westerner believes that Africans are simply suffering from the "chip on the shoulder syndrome" and are shouting racism to avoid facing the truth, he could do well to study the American response to Soviet accusations that AIDS was manufactured in an American military laboratory. These were reported in the Christmas 1986 issue of the *African Guardian:*

Predictably, the Americans have been up in arms. The articles in the Soviet media that spoke of an American origin were rebutted by American Ambassador Arthur Hartman. In one such response, he said the articles "are nothing more than a blatant and repugnant attempt to sow hatred and fear of Americans among the Soviet population and to abuse a medical tragedy affecting people all over the world, including in the Soviet Union, for base propaganda purposes." (The Soviet Union had only one case, our add).

In a summary of the ambassador's responses however, by the US information Agency, an attempt is made to mediate the conflict by ascribing origin to a neutral venue: Africa. Said the summary: "In his letter to the editor of *Literaturnaya Gazeta,* the ambassador pointed out that even Soviet scientists agree that AIDS originated in Central Africa and may have existed for several hundred or even several thousand years, or may have evolved from another virus."

Quoting Dr. Jukka Suni, a Finnish AIDS expert, an attempt is then made to impugn the reputation of Searle (a London venereologist and supporter of a laboratory origin, our add) who Jukka says is "a doctor but not a researcher."[12]

This is news to Africans, as most of the proponents of the African connection have been doctors, not researchers. Criticism of the Soviet Union has also come from the US Defence Department, reported in *Capital Gay:*

> The US Defence Department is claiming that the Soviet Union is waging a smear campaign blaming Aids on American biological warfare experiments held at army laboratories near Washington.[13]

If Africans believe that the 'African connection' is an elaborate plot to absolve America of responsibility for the AIDS epidemic, they surely cannot be accused of paranoia!

References
1.   Yinka Adeyemi. *The origin of AIDS.* Concord Weekly, July 11, 1985, p46.
2.   ibid Yinka Adeyemi.
3.   ibid Yinka Adeyemi.
4.   ibid Yinka Adeyemi.
5.   Francois Misser. *Trying to break the African Connection.* New African, January 1986, No 220 p13-4.
6.   ibid Francois Misser.
7.   ibid Francois Misser.
8.   ibid Francois Misser.
9.   Editorial, *The Herald*, Harare, Thursday April 2, 1987.
10. P Ochieng. *Africa not to blame for AIDS.* New African, January 1987, p25.
11. ibid P Ochieng.
12. *The politics of origin.* The African Guardian, December 25, 1986, p14-5.
13. *Soviet smear.* Capital Gay, London, April 24, 1987.

Chapter 12

Racism or Science?

When Western researchers descended upon central African countries, it was not at the request of African governments. To the contrary, European doctors had diagnosed AIDS in a number of patients of central African origin residing in Europe, and concluded that out there, perhaps lurking in the steaming African jungles, were thousands or even millions more. In their imaginations they conjured up some "isolated tribe" who may have harboured the virus for centuries, transmitting it to the rest of the world subsequent to the arrival of Western "civilisation".

With a singlemindedness of purpose doctors from the West arrived in Africa and set about their task. They gathered together groups of sick and dying patients, and diagnosed them as suffering from AIDS to the exclusion of all other possibilities. Without the ethical constraints that applied in their own countries, they conducted small and unreliable seroepidemiological surveys that "proved" that millions of Africans were infected with the virus. They barely paused to question, let alone explain why so few of these seropositive people showed any evidence of the disease. To prove the disease had originated in Africa they fetched old blood samples collected on previous safaris from the bottom of their freezers, and subjected them to the same unreliable tests. And then they broke the news to a Western public eager for yet another story of millions dying in Africa. This activity was not motivated by a genuine concern for Africa. The researchers claimed that identification of the source of AIDS would help find a cure and thus avert the impending catastrophe in their own countries. Only black people seemed to be asking the obvious questions: why black people, why Haiti, why Africa, when the great majority of cases were and are still occurring in North America and Western Europe?

When another sexually transmitted disease, syphilis, first appeared in Europe in the Middle Ages the English said it was a French disease. That was of course before NATO, and the English and the French were then inveterate enemies. On the other hand Tzarist Russia thought that syphilis was a Polish disease and that too was before the Warsaw Treaty. Neither assertion helped to find a cure for syphilis. In the modern world, when it comes to scapegoating our horizons have broadened greatly. Instead of blaming our next door neighbours for the problems that beset us, whole races are held responsible and villified for their sins. When AIDS first appeared amongst white American homosexuals, they were the obvious scapegoat. But the homosexuals were still Americans, and the disease was perceived as an essentially American phenomenon. Given the racist stereotyping of black people as dirty, disease carrying and sexually promiscuous, it was virtually inevitable that black people, on the first sighting of the disease amongst them, would be attributed with its source. Thus the 'gay plague' changed overnight to the 'Haitian disease'. Although the Haitian hypothesis collapsed, the idea of black people as the source of AIDS was too attractive to abandon. Attention shifted to the African continent itself. Racism, not science, motivated the search for the origin of AIDS.

Racism has been used to justify the enrichment and economic advancement of Europe at the expense of the rest of the world, and to imbue the poorer classes of Europe with a belief in their superiority by identification with a master race. But where racism was used to justify slavery it was most pernicious. To treat millions of Africans like some form of domestic animal or worse was considered acceptable because these people were thought to be really a sub-human species, more animal than human. Slavery was good for them! An illustration of this attitude was provided by Angela Davis in her book *Women, Race and Class:*

> The conditions of our problem are as follows: 1. A century or two ago the negroes were savages in the wilds of Africa. 2. Those who were brought to America, and their descendants, have acquired a certain amount of civilisation, and are now in some degree fitted for life in modern civilised society. 3. This progress of the negroes has been in very large measure the result of their association with civilised white people. 4. An immense mass of the negroes is sure to remain for an indefinite period in the midst of the civilised white nation. The problem is, how can we best provide for their peaceful residence and their further progress in this nation of white men and how best can we guard against their lapsing back into barbarism?[1]

Black people were disease ridden, dirty in their habits, uncontrolled in their sexual behaviour, and incapable of higher human values such as honesty or sexual morality. Such views were succinctly expressed by an apologist for racism, Winfield Collins, in a book published in 1918 entitled "The Truth About Lynching and the Negro in the South (In Which the Author Pleads that the South Be Made Safe for the White Race)":

> Two of the Negro's most prominent characteristics are the utter lack of chastity and complete ignorance of veracity. The Negro's sexual laxity, considered so immoral or even criminal in the white man's civilisation, may have been all but a virtue in the habitat of his origin. There, nature developed in him intense sexual passions to offset his high death rate.[2]

The use of the term "habitat" is typically racist. Other humans come from countries or continents. Black people, like animals, come from "habitats". The perception of black people as animals and not humans is a recurring racist theme. Angela Davis here describes the treatment of women slaves in America:

> In fact, in the eyes of the slaveholders, slave women were not mothers at all; they were simply instruments guaranteeing the growth of the slave labour force. They were "breeders" — animals, whose monetary value could be precisely calculated in terms of their ability to multiply their numbers.
> Since slave women were classified as "breeders" as opposed to "mothers", their infant children could be sold away from them like calves from cows. One year after the importation of Africans was halted, a South Carolina court ruled that female slaves had no legal claims whatever on their children. Consequently, according to this ruling, children could be sold away from their mothers at any age because "the young of slaves... stand on the same footing as other animals."[3]

White attitudes to black people seem to have changed little since Emancipation. A November 1986 issue of the conservative British weekly, *The Spectator,* addressed the problem of the spread of AIDS in the British heterosexual population:

> But there is another endangered group. To alert or protect them will require still more unfashionable candour than to address the homosexuals. That group is the West Indians. Their men sire their children, and often move on to another partner. Stable families are rarer than among whites, let alone Indians. To talk to West Indians about Aids will require more plain-speaking — and risk more cries of 'racism' — than has been dreamt of in Lord Whitelaw's philosophy. It will be a brave government that would do it in time. But it will probably have to be done in the end.[4]

Other humans father their children, but West Indians move from partner to partner, 'siring' their children like some stud animal.

Underlying the assumption that West Indians will require "more plain-speaking" than the rest of the population is the belief that they are both more stupid and less able to control their sexuality than other Britons. In fact more plain speaking, it would seem, is required for the entire heterosexual British population. According to a report in *The Guardian* of 6th June 1987, an international Aids conference in Washington was told that the Government's £10 million campaign of newspaper and television advertisements and pamphlets had failed so far to make heterosexuals modify their behaviour.

According to racist mythology, "darkest" Africa was some vast, impenetrable jungle inhabited by humans living Tarzan-like in close cohabitation with monkeys, devoid of history and the rudiments of civilisation. Even eminent British historians such as Hugh Trevor-Roper, now Lord Dacre (of the Hitler diaries fame), regard sub-Saharan Africa as outside the scope of human history:

> Undergraduates, seduced, as always, by the changing breath of journalistic fashion, demand that they should be taught the history of black Africa. Perhaps, in the future, there will be some African history to teach. But at present there is none, or very little: there is only the history of the Europeans in Africa. The rest is largely darkness, like the history of pre-European, pre-Columbian America. And darkness is not a subject for history.
>
> Please do not misunderstand me. I do not deny that men existed even in dark countries and dark centuries... If all history is equal, as some now believe, there is no reason why we should study one section of it rather than another; for certainly we cannot study it all. Then indeed we may neglect our own history and amuse ourselves with the unrewarding gyrations of barbarous tribes in picturesque but irrelevant corners of the globe...
>
> It is European techniques, European examples, European ideas which have shaken the non-European world out of its past — out of barbarism in Africa, out of a far older, slower, more majestic civilization in Asia; and the history of the world, for the last five centuries, in so far as it has significance, has been European history.[5]

Presumably he is referring to the history of slavery, genocide and wholescale plunder. Such were the benefits of European civilisation! According to such racist views, the only form of social organisation that existed in Africa prior to European penetration was the "tribe". These "tribes" were lacking any complex social organisation, had no experience of settled community life, and were constantly at war with eachother. Such an erroneous view precludes any appreciation of the complexity of cultures, languages, and nationalities with different forms of political and social organisation that existed prior to colonisation, and their transformation into the modern nation states of the post colonial era.

With preconceived notions of a barbarous mass of people living in primitive conditions, Westerners seem only capable of perceiving negative aspects of African society which they inevitably attribute to the corruption and inefficiency of African governments. Western doctors researching AIDS in Africa frequently criticise poor medical facilities in African countries. Such criticisms, often unjustified, do not take into consideration the parlous state of the health services bequeathed by the departing colonial powers, and the substantial achievements of independent governments to redress these deficiencies. Walter Rodney, the late Guyanese historian, illustrated this point most clearly:

> For the first three decades of colonialism, hardly anything was done that could remotely be termed a service to the African people. It was in fact only after the last war that social services were built as a matter of policy. How little they amounted to does not really need illustrating. After all, the statistics which show that Africa today is underdeveloped are the statistics representing the state of affairs at the end of colonialism. For that matter, the figures at the end of the first decade of African independence in spheres such as health, housing and education are often several times higher than the figures inherited by the newly independent governments.[6]

Zambia provides one of many such examples. Under British colonial rule there were only three general hospitals, mostly catering for whites. A Zambian Government publication outlined the changes since independence:

> Immediately after Independence, the new Government and the Ministry of Health realised the lack of adequate medical facilities in the country. Programmes were drawn up for expansion of medical care throughout the country. Today, ten years after Independence the expansion and planning is still going on. Under the Ten Year National Plan 1972-1981 the main objective is to provide an integrated curative and preventive health service to all the people of Zambia...
>
> District hospitals, staffed by medical officers, registered nurses and auxiliary staff, are responsible for the health care of the entire district and for the supervision of health centers and sub-centers.
>
> At provincial level there is a general hospital headed by a medical superintendent and staffed by some specialists as well as general duty medical officers, and offering major surgery and other specialist services. There are nine hospitals — seven of them at provincial headquarters and the other two at Choma and Mbala...
>
> There are three central hospitals — at Lusaka, Kitwe and Ndola — and these provide the widest range of specialist services in the country...

In March, 1973, the first group of 13 doctors graduated from the School
of Medicine of the University of Zambia. Although the number is small,
the occasion is a milestone in the history of the development of health
services in this country... Scholarships are offered to Zambian doctors to
train in various specialist fields abroad...

A health services training school complex is to be established at Ndola
for the training of 200 registered nurses and 50 midwives. There will also
be training both for X-ray and laboratory assistants. The building project
is to be financed by a World Bank Loan.[7]

In Zimbabwe, achievements in education and health have also
been impressive:

Education has been one of the areas of greatest Government achievement
since Independence. In a very short time Zimbabwe has been able to
outstrip the record of most of its neighbours in terms of the provision of
education facilities. As a result primary education has literally trebled
from an enrolment of 819,586 in 1979 to over 2.1 million in 1984.
Secondary education has increased sixfold from 66,215 in 1979 to 422,584
in 1984.[8]

And from *The Guardian*, 17th April, 1986:

The country's health service record is impressive; almost 4,500 health
workers have been trained since independence, 450 war-damaged clinics
and over 200 health centers completed by 1986 at a cost of over Z$17.50
millions.[9]

It is hardly surprising that Africans are offended when doctors from
the former colonial powers criticise their 'inadequate health services'.
Even in Zaire, health services under the Mobutu dictatorship are
better than anything the Belgian colonialists provided.

Underlying all such judgements of Africa and Africans are opposite
assumptions of Western conditions and behaviour. Africans are
considered promiscuous "by Western standards" — by whose
standards, one wonders. Africans would find it difficult to match the
pace of some leading British politicians who resigned following
scandals involving prostitutes. Can we accuse Africans of tribalism
whilst ignoring the internecine struggles of various nationalist and
separatist groups in Europe? Although, of course, such conflicts are
not considered tribal outside Africa, and euphemistic terms such as
'communal', 'new nationalist' and 'religious' are used. And could the
horrors of the Second World War in Europe be considered to result
from some inherently barbaric streak in the European personality?

The extermination of millions in the concentration camps of Europe
during World War II, the post-war anti-colonial struggles, the
campaigns for civil rights for Black people in the United States and
recently the struggle to end Apartheid in South Africa have all

contributed to a greater awareness in the West of the inherent evils of racism. One response to racism came in the fourth UNESCO (United Nations Educational Scientific and Cultural Organisation) *Statement on Race,* drafted in Paris in 1967:

> Racial prejudice and discrimination in the world today arise from historical and social phenomena and falsely claim the sanction of science. It is, therefore, the responsibility of all biological and social scientists, philosophers, and others working in related disciplines, to ensure that the results of their research are not misused by those who wish to propagate racial prejudice and encourage discrimination.[10]

Yet any awareness of racism seems to have bypassed the medical scientists and journalists almost entirely. Medical textbooks and journals remain littered with racist references and terminology such as "civilised peoples", "negroes" and "bantus" long abandoned elsewhere. Indeed a historian from the Centre of African Studies at Edinburgh University, criticising the historical accuracy of a recent article in *The Lancet* about the relationship between salt intake and hypertension in West Africa, made the following comments:

> What dismayed me, however, about Wilson's article was his statement that "medical researchers" still have a "long-standing convention of classifying man into racial groups for research purposes". Well, it is now some thirty years since what I had always supposed was the last bastion of racial medical theory — the belief that sickle cell genes are found only in members of the "Negro race" — was exploded (when they were discovered among Indians, Turks and Italians, and found almost absent among the Kru of West Africa).[11]

It is striking that the scientists who most consistently avoid racist generalisations come from Germany and South Africa, countries infamous for their racial chauvinism. Where racism is or has been elevated to the position of official government policy, its manifestations are perhaps more readily appreciated and avoided by those who wish to preserve their scientific integrity.

It was hardly surprising, indeed almost inevitable, that the source and transmission of a new and deadly sexually transmitted disease would be attributed to black people whatever the evidence. When the researchers grudgingly accepted that Haitians had been infected by Americans, other black people were sought out to be similarly (dis)credited. The original proposal of the "old disease of Africa" was untenable from conception. As many African scientists pointed out, there were extensive contacts for many centuries between different African peoples, and between Africa and the rest of the world, and the disease would surely have been seen in Europe long before it appeared in white homosexuals on the west coast of the

United States. Apart from such historical considerations (and some Western researchers are extraordinarily ignorant of African history) no scientific evidence could be found to support the "Old African" origin hypothesis. Yet this hypothesis gained widespread acceptance as theory and even fact in Western scientific circles. To resolve these contradictions, the scientists conveniently reduced the time scale for the onset of AIDS in humans from centuries to decades or less, and the "old disease" hypothesis was simply transferred from African humans to African monkeys. To "prove" that AIDS appeared in central Africa before the United States, patients in Africa with wasting diseases were retrospectively diagnosed as AIDS without substantial evidence. Additional "proof" was provided by unreliable tests conducted on 25 year-old blood samples. The African green monkey was singled out as the source of the precursor of the AIDS virus, although a number of other animal viruses, such as the Visna virus in Icelandic sheep are equally if not more likely candidates. All this fitted in very nicely with the belief that Africans were both evolutionarily and physically closer to monkeys than people elsewhere in the world.

If the minds of the scientists were not so confused by racist preconceptions, they would have appreciated the contradictions and downright absurdity of many of their conclusions. A plethora of explanations were offered for the high rates of seropositivity amongst Africans in rural areas who showed no evidence of AIDS: that Africans were immune to HIV, that because the virus had been present in the population for a long time, the virus had reached a natural equilibrium, and so on. The issue of the reliability of the ELISA test could have been settled by crosschecking with different tests such as indirect immunofluoresence prior to publication of the results. But scientists already convinced that Africans were riddled with AIDS were unlikely to question the validity of their findings. When a few researchers showed that the seroepidemiological results were unreliable, their findings were greeted with little comment and were largely ignored. The appearance of AIDS amongst wealthy city dwellers but not rural peasants provoked even more convoluted explanations of immunological differences between the two populations. Such hypotheses fly in the face of the demographic reality of large population shifts from rural to urban areas since colonial times, obvious even to the casual observer let alone a social scientist or historian. Other areas of contradiction avoided by the scientists were the low or absent incidence of AIDS in student and immigrant African populations in the socialist countries and Britain, and the declining proportion of African cases elsewhere in Europe. This hardly squares with an epidemic raging through the African continent.

The unquestioned belief in the extraordinarily high rate of HIV infection led to a host of speculations about African sexual behaviour completely unsupported by any evidence. Africans were said to indulge in anal intercourse and intercourse during menstruation, and were far more promiscuous than other people. Indeed the alleged rate of HIV infection in central Africa is much higher than the rate of other far more infectious sexually transmitted diseases such as gonorrhea and syphilis, an issue never taken up by the researchers. If claims that a third of sexually active adults in some central African countries are infected with AIDS are true, life in these countries must be one endless orgy.

Because scientists found it so difficult to imagine that white people could infect Africans with AIDS and not the reverse, such a possibility has never been seriously investigated. If, as the researchers proposed, AIDS had originated in some obscure rural area but appeared in the cities because of greater urban sexual promiscuity, then it surely would have first appeared amongst the most promiscuous urban Africans, 'low class' female prostitutes and their clients, poor male workers. Instead, AIDS first appeared amongst educated Africans with a history of foreign travel. As a study in Kenya revealed, this group frequented 'high class' prostitutes whose clientele also included foreign tourists and businessmen. This is an obvious route for the entry of AIDS into Africa, but the scientists seem to avoid any such interpretation, preferring to juggle their figures to 'prove' the virus was travelling along 'traditional trade routes' from the centre to the coast, rather than the opposite direction.

The possibility of a homosexual importation of AIDS into Africa is also completely ignored. For example, leading AIDS researchers such as Peter Piot fail to consider the possibility that a Belgian homosexual who had multiple partners in Zaire, Europe and Brazil may have introduced rather than contracted AIDS in Zaire.[12] African homosexuality is considered largely irrelevant by western researchers, but the role of frequently bisexual African male prostitutes in the spread of AIDS in Africa remains virtually uninvestigated. Two of the earliest Kenyan cases were bachelors, unusual in a society where social pressure to marry is intense. Two early Zambian cases "admitted single episodes of homosexual behaviour, but both had happened after the onset of symptoms of KS". There is little tolerance of homosexual behaviour in most African societies, and homosexuals are likely to be well closeted. In Europe, where homosexuality is legalised and more tolerated, there are quite a few cases of African homosexuals with AIDS.[13] Of course they have been placed in the African, and not the homosexual "at risk" category, even when they have been resident in Europe for many years. (An example is a 43-year-old Ghanaian resident in West Germany for 17 years.) Assumptions about the absence of homosexual transmission in Africa may not be well founded.

The selective bias of the AIDS researchers is reminiscent of the old comedy routine, where the comedian searches for a lost coin where the street lights are brightest, not on the dark side of the street where the coin was dropped. If the scientists only look for the origin of AIDS in Africa, they certainly will not find it anywhere else. If they had decided, because of some preconceived notion, that AIDS had originated in Aboriginal Indian tribes in Venezuela, seroepidemological studies would have shown the same high rate of false positivity, and the appearance of AIDS amongst urban Venezuelans would be 'proof' the disease had travelled from rural areas to the cities. With careful selection of the evidence and a juggling of statistics, it is possible to prove anything 'scientifically' — that the world is flat, that there are fairies in the bottom of the garden. But science is not about careful selection of data. It is about searching for all possible explanations that fit **all** the known facts.

The widespread, uncritical acceptance of the AIDS from Africa hypothesis by the normally sceptical scientific community is most disturbing. It would be comforting to believe that this was a simple mistake or an unfortunate result of an excess of enthusiasm. It seems to us far more likely that the AIDS researchers, the medical "experts", the media and the public at large are affected by the insidious and frequently unrecognised disease of racism. Let us hope that the truth now prevails.

References
1. Quoted in Angela Davis. *Women, Race and Class.* Notes, Chapter 1, item 1.
2. ibid p180-1.
3. ibid p7.
4. *How to stop a plague.* The Spectator, November 8, 1986, P5.
5. Hugh Trevor Roper. *The rise of christian Europe.* Thames Hudson, 1966, p9-11.
6. W Rodney. *How Europe underdeveloped Africa.* Bogle-L'Ouverture Publications, 1983, p224.
7. *A decade of achievement.* Zambian Government publication, 1974, p37-9.

8.   *Achievements and problems in education since Independence.* The Journal on Social Change and Development, No 10, 1985, p10.
9.   *The Guardian*, April 17, 1986.
10. Quoted from Ruth Benedict. *Race and Racism.* Routledge and Kegan Paul, 1983, p185-6.
11. C Fyfe. *Past salt supplies in west Africa and blood pressures today.* The Lancet, May 24, 1986, p1218.
12. R Colebunders, H Taelman, P Piot. *Acquired immunodeficiency syndrome (AIDS) in Africa.* Tropical Doctor, January 1985, p9-12.
13. *Acquired immune deficiency syndrome (AIDS). Report on the situation in Europe as of 30 June, 1985.* WHO Weekly Epidemiological Record No 40, October 4, 1985, p305-12.

Postscript (1989)

In this book we have attempted a critical assessment of the "science" that has sought to place Africa at the centre of the worldwide AIDS epidemic. In the two years since the book's first publication, it has been gratifying to find that much of the evidence for an African origin for the Human Immunodeficiency Virus (HIV) has not stood the test of time.[1,2] Most importantly, the African green monkey is generally now no longer thought to harbour a precursor to HIV that crossed the species barrier,[3–7] and other animal viruses, particularly retroviruses in sheep and cattle, are under consideration.[8–10] Alternative hypotheses are beginning to appear in the mainstream scientific literature, in particular the possibility of a laboratory origin.[11] There seems to be widespread acceptance that the early seroepidemiological studies were misleading,[12,13] and there is also evidence that the supposed early African cases that predated the American epidemic were not AIDS, although this information has not been published in the literature.

Although the scientific evidence for an African origin has been found wanting, the scientists are only reluctantly abandoning their favourite hypothesis and are considering the alternatives with little enthusiasm. Now that AIDS researchers are no longer able to present the African hypothesis with conviction, we are told that the origin of AIDS is no longer important and that efforts should be directed at containing the epidemic. However, if a laboratory origin is a possibility, then surely the issue is of great importance for avoiding further new and deadly epidemics. If the AIDS epidemic did not originate in Africa, then the routes by which the virus is spreading to Africa need investigation. Yet issues such as the importation of blood products from the West, for example, have been almost completely ignored, and Western sex tourism has been considered as a route for AIDS transmission only from Africa to the West. Indeed, Western AIDS researchers, now claiming with little evidence that their blood tests are reliable, are ever more insistent that millions of Africans are already infected and are a major route by which AIDS will spread to the heterosexual population of the West.[14,15,16]

Perhaps the most important reasons for the reluctance to face the truth about AIDS in Africa are more political than scientific. When the "African epidemic" is so grossly exaggerated, the enormous scale of the epidemic in the United States is proportionally diminished. Moreover, if Africans are supposedly dying by the millions, then it becomes politically acceptable to use them as a vast human laboratory for testing an AIDS vaccine. Such are the potential consequences of unsubstantiated reports in the mass media (as in BBC TV news on World AIDS Day, December 1 1988) claiming that there are "an estimated 149,000 AIDS cases in Africa".

A end to the monkey business?

A body blow has now been dealt to the notion that the AIDS virus originated in central Africa. An AIDS-like virus in monkeys was supposed to have jumped the species barrier when Africans variously ate monkeys, were bitten by them, or gave their children dead monkeys as pets, or perhaps when they injected monkey blood as a sexual stimulant. Such absurd notions were given scientific credibility by two Harvard researchers, Essex and Kanki, who reported that they had isolated an AIDS-like virus from wild caught African green monkeys (see page 72).

Their research was exposed in March 1988, when Essex and Kanki had to admit that the virus they claimed to have isolated from wild caught African green monkeys was a laboratory contaminant.[17–20] This came to light when other researchers tried unsuccessfully to repeat the Essex and Kanki experiments on wild African green monkeys. Subsequently the genetic sequence of the macaque and green monkey viruses, and of another supposedly human virus called HTLV–IV, were found to be identical. The alleged African monkey precursor of the human AIDS virus was none other than the virus that had been causing an AIDS-like illness in macaque monkeys in primate research laboratories in the United States. The origin of the macaque virus is obscure, as it does not infect wild macaque monkeys but does have some similarity with the human AIDS viruses, particularly the more recently isolated HIV-2.[21]

The Guardian of March 8 1988 reported these findings in an article titled "Don't blame Africa yet", written by none other than Renée

Sabatier from the Panos Institute. As the title of the article suggested, the scientists were still doing their best:

> But there is more research in the wings that could yet keep the green monkey theory alive. Independently of Kanki and Essex, at least three other groups of scientists, in Japan, Germany and the US, say that they have isolated an Aids-like virus from wild and captive African green monkeys.[22]

Those who wanted to blame Africa were to be sadly disappointed. The findings of the Japanese researchers were published in *Nature* in June 1988.[23] The virus isolated from African green monkeys bore little resemblance to either the macaque virus or the human AIDS viruses. Carel Mulder, Professor of Pharmacology, Molecular Genetics and Microbiology at the University of Massachusetts Medical School, made the following comment:

> The fact that the SIV_{agm} sequence is so remarkably different from the human AIDS viruses indicates that the human viruses cannot have originated from African green monkeys in recent times, as had been predicted by many people.[24]

It is difficult to understand why this virus was called an African green monkey Simian Immunodeficiency Virus, as it does not cause immunodeficiency in African green monkeys. We are left to wonder about the origin of the virus that causes an AIDS-like illness in captive macaque monkeys but does not occur in wild monkeys. Did this virus originate in a laboratory? Could it be the true precursor of the human AIDS virus?

For anyone who still has illusions about the objectivity of science or the integrity of some AIDS researchers, it is instructive to read the October 1988 issue of *Scientific American*, devoted to AIDS. The section titled "The origins of the AIDS virus", written by Essex and Kanki, was illustrated with a full-page colour picture of an African green monkey. Eight months after admitting that the African green monkey virus was a laboratory contaminant, Essex and Kanki had the audacity to claim that the laboratory macaque virus was isolated from wild African green monkeys:

> Why SIV is endemic in these wild African monkeys but seems to do them no harm, and is also found in the captive Asian macaques, where it causes disease, was (and still is) an enigma . . .[25]

Of course the article did not mention any alternative hypotheses, such as a possible Euro-American[26] or laboratory origin[27,28] for HIV. Nor did it mention the genetic similarities between the human immunodeficiency virus and the Visna virus of sheep or the bovine immunodeficiency virus of cattle.[29–31]

The isolation of a second human retrovirus, HIV-2, from West African patients was reported in 1986.[32] The incidence of AIDS in West Africa is low[33] and is largely confined to prostitutes who work in areas frequented by foreign tourists.[34] Until the work of Kanki and Essex was discredited, there was much speculation that HIV-2 had also evolved in Africa and was the missing link in the transmission of AIDS from monkeys to humans.[35] If, as research now suggests, there is no closely related monkey virus ancestor for HIV except in monkeys in American laboratories, what is the origin of HIV-2? According to a report in *New Scientist* of the 1988 Stockholm AIDS conference,

> Researchers are finding that the human immunodeficiency virus is far more genetically variable than once supposed. Individuals can be infected with several unique strains of HIV. Some babies of infected women are born with quite different strains of HIV than those found in their mothers. A single infected cell can harbour as many as seven genetic variants of HIV . . .
>
> The current method – growing the virus through several generations in strains of cultured human cells – tends to select artificially for certain strains of HIV that grow well in culture . . .[36]

The place of HIV-2 in this viral heterogeneity is far from clear.

An "old disease" revisited

Although African green monkeys have now been largely discredited as the source of the AIDS epidemic, some AIDS researchers still cling hopefully to the notion of the "old disease from Africa". Kevin De Cock, one of the earliest proponents of this idea, recently published an article titled "The prevalence of infection with human immunodeficiency virus over a 10-year period in rural Zaire":

> In 1985 we tested 659 human serum samples, collected in the remote Equater province of Zaire in 1976, for antibody to human immunodeficiency virus (HIV). Five (0.8 percent) were positive, and HIV was isolated from one of these. Follow-up investigations in 1985 revealed that three of the five seropositive persons had died of illnesses suggestive of acquired immunodeficiency syndrome (AIDS), and two remained healthy but seropositive. In 1986, a serosurvey we conducted using a cluster-sampling technique in the same region showed a seroprevalence of 0.8 percent in 389 randomly selected residents . . . We believe that the long-term stability of HIV infection in residents of rural Zaire suggests that social change may have promoted the spread of AIDS in Africa.[37]

Ninety people who were seronegative in 1976 were traced in 1985 and 1986, and all remained seronegative.

The authors describe Equater province as "remote" but provide us with a map showing that the villages where the study took place were alongside the river Zaire, between the capital, Kinshasa, and Kisangani. The river Zaire has been a major centre for trade (including slave trading) in central Africa for centuries,[38] so it is absurd to suggest that a sexually transmitted disease could have remained isolated in Equater province until the 1970s. The samples were tested with ELISA and Western blot. Moreover, the combined false positive rate for the two tests is assumed to be zero, but this is unlikely even for samples taken in the West and is improbable for stored African serum. Patients with infectious diseases are more likely to give a false positive result than healthy subjects, and it cannot even be assumed that all seropositive patients who died of illnesses resembling AIDS were actually suffering from that disease. Virus was isolated from only one subject, a "free woman" who had lived in Kinshasa from 1972 to 1976 and died in 1978 of an AIDS-like illness. This is said to be the earliest HIV isolate.[39] However, a 15-year-old American boy died of an AIDS-like illness in 1969, and his tissues have subsequently been reported to contain HIV antigen.[40] In 1977 Kaposi's sarcoma was reported in two American homosexuals who were later diagnosed as suffering from AIDS, and these patients were probably infected in the early 1970s.[41]

Sexual activity and blood products are two obvious routes for transmission of HIV into the Zairean population by the mid 1970s. Luc Montagnier has suggested that HIV may have been introduced to Zaire by the UN Peace-keeping Corps in the 1960s,[42] but there has also been a substantial expatriate presence, mostly American and Belgian, in Zaire since that time. Indeed, if HIV had been present in Zaire in the 1960s, it is difficult to understand why the disease did not spread to the Irish, Indian, Swedish and Ghanaian troops that comprised the UN Corps, but instead first appeared in the United States. After all the discussion about African promiscuity and abnormal sexual practices, it is extraordinary that Equater province seems to be the only place in the world where HIV seropositivity has not risen in a ten-year period. Either Africans are less promiscuous than the rest of humankind, or the reported results represent false seropositivity. In either case it would seem that rural Africans, who comprise the great majority of the African population, will not, after all, die by the million.

Early African non-cases, and some early Euro-American cases?

One of the most cited papers in support of an African origin for AIDS, "AIDS in a Danish surgeon (Zaire, 1976)", described the case

143

of a surgeon who had supposedly caught HIV from her patients whilst working in a hospital in Equater province.[43] An illustration of how questionable science can be translated into popular mythology can be found in the best-selling book by Randy Shilts, *And the Band Played On*, about the AIDS epidemic. Under "Dramatis Personae" he listed her as "Danish surgeon in Zaire, first Westerner documented to have died of AIDS". He described her work in Zaire in a most melodramatic fashion:

> The battle between humans and disease was nowhere more bitterly fought than here in the fetid equatorial climate, where heat and humidity fuel the generation of new life forms . . . Here, on the frontiers of the world's harshest medical realities, Grethe Rask tended the sick . . .[44]

A British researcher, Dr Janie Grote, wrote to Dr Bygbjerg, the author of the paper about the Danish surgeon, inquiring further about Dr Rask, and received the following reply:

> We have found a very small serum sample, which was taken shortly before the patient died in 1977, and we know already that it was HIV-I ELISA antibody negative. Thus, we cannot prove that the patient had AIDS, although the clinical picture was very suggestive . . . Personally I think that she was infected (if at all by HIV) during her work as a surgeon in northern Zaire . . .[45]

So this famous AIDS case was seronegative. This information has not, of course, been presented in the scientific literature, and Bygbjerg's article continues to lead the citation index of cases "proving" an African origin for AIDS.

Another early case of AIDS was of a British woman who was supposed to have caught AIDS from her Ghanaian ex-husband, who, without any evidence, was considered an AIDS carrier (see page 27):

> It must be assumed that the husband is an asymptomatic carrier and himself contracted HTLV-III infection in Zambia, where there is evidence of an AIDS-like epidemic.

The man was eventually traced and tested for HIV; ELISA, Western blot and radioimmunoprecipitation tests were all negative.[46] In Britain the Communicable Disease Surveillance Centre at Colindale categorises patients with HIV infection according to the continent where the infection originated.[47] How Colindale arrives at such conclusions remains a mystery, as promiscuous people who travel are unlikely to confine their sexual activity to any one continent. Presumably this British woman has been reported as acquiring her infection from Africa, and one wonders just how many more of these cases are similarly attributed without substantiation.

Most Western AIDS researchers have been preoccupied with AIDS-like cases with an African connection to the exclusion of similar cases in America or Europe. In a paper published in 1987 titled "Evidence for a Euro-American origin of human immunodeficiency virus", 28 patients who died of AIDS-like illnesses before the onset of the AIDS epidemic were presented:

> Using disseminated Kaposi's sarcoma as a probable marker of AIDS, 28 cases (25 men) were reported from 1902 to 1966. Mean age of patients was 42 years, and all died in less than two-and-a-half years. Six had signs compatible with opportunistic infections and one had disseminated tuberculosis.
>
> Significant sociocultural changes occurred in the male homosexual community during the 1970s, reflected by significant increases in sexually transmitted diseases. The incidence of hepatitis B tripled in this population from 1970 to 1980 and was then first associated with transmission by anal intercourse. These changes could have brought an endemic, sporadically expressed virus to epidemic proportions, allowing for the subsequent recognition of AIDS as a clinical entity . . .[48]

The earlier cases were reported from Europe, and most of the later cases came from North America. The patients were mostly younger males, and the symptoms were very suggestive of AIDS:

> The spectrum of symptoms in these patients included weakness, anorexia, melena, fever, night sweats, dyspnea, diarrhea, and in one patient with central nervous system Kaposi's sarcoma, focal seizures . . .
>
> In 1940 Hansson stated that Kaposi's sarcoma was more aggressive in the younger patient, yet gave no support for this. Not until 1959, when Cox and Helwig published their summary of Kaposi's sarcoma, were patients evaluated at the Armed Forces Institute of Pathology and the young age of patients was noted. Seven of the 11 patients who had died of Kaposi's sarcoma were less than age 45 years. Of these, the three who died in less than six months were all in their 20s. Tedeschi et al commented that lymph node enlargement could be an early manifestation of the disease, preceding the cutaneous lesions. He pointed out that in a number of cases the nodes revealed a "nonspecific hyperplasia" without evidence of the tumour.[49]

Abandoning the African origin, or white man speaking with forked tongue?

The origin of AIDS was discussed by a number of leading researchers at the second international conference on AIDS in Africa, held in Naples in October 1987:

> Luc Montagnier . . . the first scientist to isolate the virus that causes AIDS, agrees that if an isolated population in Africa existed as a reservoir

for the virus, researchers would probably have found it by now. The data suggesting that the virus comes from Africa are weak, Montagnier said . . . "The evidence [for HIV-I originating in Africa] is very weak . . ." he told the conference. "Maybe we should look at another part of the world."[50]

Jonathan Mann, the director of the WHO AIDS programme, also felt obliged to distance himself from an African origin:

The World Health Organisation's position is that there is not yet enough information about the origin of the virus. There are absolutely no data to support any hypothesis, according to Dr Jonathan Mann, director of WHO's special programme on AIDS.

"The more information that emerges, the less we know about where this virus came from, how long it has been in the world, and how it grew to become the problem that it is today," he said.

The syndrome has too often unveiled thinly disguised prejudices about race, religion, sex, social class, and nationality, and the Africans properly resent that Africa has been singled out, Dr Mann said. If San Francisco was accused of being the original source of HIV with no more proof than there is that Africa is the source, special interest groups would be up in arms, he said . . .

Dr Mann said nothing will keep people from coming up with "cheap hypotheses" about the origin of AIDS. "They die a natural death when no subsequent evidence develops to take them seriously. But perhaps journals should have a special page for them labeled 'fuzzy ideas'," he said.

The real danger is that future authors might use such discredited, but published, hypotheses as scientific references for future articles, he said.[51]

This would seem a classic case of white man speaking with forked tongue, as papers by Jonathan Mann himself or Peter Piot et al would be prime candidates for any such "fuzzy ideas" column. Indeed, where has Jonathan Mann, the director of the World Health Organisation's AIDS programme, ever criticised the racist nonsense published in the medical journals or the mass media, except at conferences attended by Africans? Did he or any other Western AIDS researcher, for example, complain to *The Lancet* about the lettter published there in June 1987?

Sir, – The isolation from monkeys of retroviruses closely related to HIV strongly suggests a simian origin for this virus . . . Several unlikely hypotheses have been put forward to explain the indirect transmission of the virus from monkey to man – for example, the theory that the disease spread to man through bites or the cutting up and consumption of monkey meat or the arthropod vector hypothesis. In his book on the sexual life of people in the Great Lakes area of Africa, Kashamura writes: "pour stimuler intense, on leur inocule dans les cuisses, la région du pubis et le dos du sang prélevé sur un singe, pour un homme, sur une guenon, pour une femme" (to stimulate a man or a woman and induce them to intense sexual activity, monkey blood [for a man] or she-monkey blood [for a woman] was directly inoculated in the pubic area and also in the thighs and back). These magic practices would therefore constitute an efficient experimental transmission model and could be responsible for the emergence of AIDS in man.[52]

This theory came in for particular derision at the Naples conference:

When queried regarding the plausibility of a premise put forth in a letter to *The Lancet* suggesting that a bizarre tribal ritual of injecting monkey blood into the pubic region of young African men and women to stimulate intense sexual activity could be responsible for the emergence of AIDS in man, researchers from Zaire, Congo, and Belgium were unanimous in declaring it to be preposterous . . .[53]

Scientific racism

Although many Western AIDS researchers now appreciate that they have offended and angered many black people, they remain ignorant of their unconscious racism and continue to cause offence. The September 1988 edition of *Medicine International* was devoted to the subject of AIDS, and as usual there was an article on AIDS in Africa, but no similar discussion about AIDS in any other continent. The authors were Paul Nunn and Keith McAdam, clinical lecturer and professor respectively at the London School of Hygiene and Tropical Medicine. Paul Nunn's experience of Africa was confined to a short period in the Gambia, a country with a low incidence of AIDS; this was rather more than his colleague's, as Professor McAdam has never worked in Africa at all but spent three years in New Guinea and nine years at the National Institutes of Health, where Gallo and company also conduct their research. They comment on the problems created by the earlier AIDS research in Africa:

Initial claims that the disease had been present in Africa for long enough for widespread immunity to have developed in exposed populations were false; epidemics of AIDS were as new in Africa as elsewhere. Considerable damage has been done to international research collaboration as a result of these claims.[54]

But later in the same article they add insult to injury:

The scale of the African AIDS epidemic has led to speculation that heterosexual transmission is more efficient in Africa than elsewhere . . . Social and cultural factors, such as the African tradition of male sexual freedom, may also play a part. The circulation of myths such as the only

147

cure for AIDS being to have sex with a virgin is likely to have a greater effect on transmission in Africa than in developed countries.[55]

What do these two gentlemen know about African traditions of male sexual freedom? If they are seriously suggesting that a significant number of African men with AIDS are having sex with virgins, then on what evidence? Are scientific journals the place for European fantasies about primitive tribal rituals of virgin sacrifice? Let it be clearly noted that leading academics at the London School of Hygiene and Tropical Medicine believe that Africans are more promiscuous and prone to irrational beliefs than the rest of humanity. Perhaps the staff at the London School should undertake a course in the sociology of the sexual attitudes and behaviour of men in the United Kingdom before commenting about the behaviour of others; some racism-awareness training would also not go amiss. It is hardly surprising that Paul Nunn works with the Panos Institute,[56] which has spread disinformation about AIDS in Africa. Towards the end of the issue of *Medicine International*, the authors provide the following advice to those about to travel to Africa:

> The most important precaution is to avoid casual sexual contact.[57]

So presumably casual sex is safe elsewhere in the world! One wonders why the British government spent millions of pounds persuading its citizens to avoid such activities back home.

A sister institution, the Liverpool School of Tropical Medicine, is prone to similar prejudices, according to the British anti-fascist monthly, *Searchlight*:

> The Liverpool School of Tropical Medicine needs major anti-racist surgery, according to a new watchdog group campaigning against racism and what it describes as a colonialist set-up at the school . . .
>
> Although 60 percent of the school's intake is from the "developing world", the mentality still seems to be that Western experts know best, and this is reflected in the curriculum, and the stereotypical and patronising material presented to students about the Third World . . . It has also failed to speak out against racialist populist thinking on the relationship between AIDS and Africa.[58]

Other AIDS researchers have recognized that their past activities have caused problems. The *British Medical Bulletin* of January 1988, titled "AIDS and HIV infection: the wider perspective", was edited by three notable exponents of the African connection, Anthony Pinching, Robin Weiss and David Miller. It reported:

> In the case of some early studies in Africa, techniques were used that had not been sufficiently well validated for African sera, given the prevalent

hypergammaglobulinaemia and a notorious tendency to "stickiness" and false positive reactions in antiglobulin assays. The observations derived from these studies have led to some confusion and have also tended to damage the credibility of foreign scientists working in Africa – especially among local leaders. Additional problems have been created when investigators have spent a short time collecting sera and basic data in a developing country, often with little guidance from local investigators, and then published the data without reference to the original context. This has tended to produce scientific data that have not been adequately placed in an anthropological perspective. Even worse, it has led to denial and resentment, jeopardising essential and potentially fruitful collaboration between investigators in the developed and developing world in the study of an issue of mutual concern. This has been particularly damaging when the pursuit has apparently been the origin of AIDS and HIV, an essentially academic question, however interesting. Such investigations have often been taken to imply blame on the region that appears to be the source. Although they were certainly never intended to impugn any community in this way, it is not difficult to see how such perceptions arose.[59]

As we have mentioned earlier in the book (page 116), Dr Pinching published "research" showing that central Africans were genetically susceptible to AIDS. His paper brought forth the following reply from a Ghanaian physician, Dr Konotey-Ahulu:

Sir, – In their paper on group-specific phenotypes and human immunodeficiency virus (HIV) infection, Dr Eales and colleagues state: "It is of interest that in an area where HIV infection is very common – namely in some parts of central Africa – the Gc If allele predominates in the indigenous population", and they cite Constans et al. On May 3 one of the authors of this paper was interviewed on the BBC World Service's "Science in Action" about their research which "may explain why the epidemic has spread faster in central Africa than even in the United States". The whole interview sounded as if a fact about central Africa had been discovered, yet it concluded with the statement "We have not yet tested this hypothesis ourselves about central Africa". So Eales et al used the data of Constans et al, which are not about AIDS-afflicted central Africa at all but about a group of pygmies (in whom AIDS is notable for its absence) and about the Peuhl Fula in Senegal, where AIDS is not much of a problem. Yet they broadcast to the world and leave the impression that there is something genetically wrong with central Africans, hence their plight vis-à-vis AIDS. The Bi-Aka pygmies, 267 of whom were described by Constans et al . . . form a tiny group of at most 60,000 pygmies in the former Central African "Empire" with a total population of 2,700,000. To use genetic data from this anthropologically distinct group, who do not even have AIDS, to cover "central Africa" leaves a lot to be desired.[60]

After this communication *The Lancet* published 8 more from researchers worldwide who repeated the work but failed to confirm that the hereditary Gc phenotype had anything to do with susceptibility to AIDS.

With this track record, and the confession that AIDS research had caused offence, we would expect the three editors of the *British Medical Bulletin* to have mended their ways. Instead, we read (on page 58):

> HIV infection appears to have spread over much of the world during the decade 1976–1986, mirroring on a larger scale the spread of its most obvious predecessor, syphilis, in Europe in the 1490s. As with early syphilis, the international spread of AIDS has led to a process of attribution and denial about the origin of the disease. However, it seems most likely that HIV spread to the United States from Africa, perhaps via Haiti, in the mid 1970s, and from the United States to many Western countries in the late 1970s and early 1980s.[61]

It is hard to believe that this was published in 1988. AIDS travelled from Africa to Haiti to the United States and then to Europe! Later in the *Bulletin*, in a section by Peter Piot and Michel Carael, we come to some more familiar territory:

> However, officially reported figures to the World Health Organisation (WHO) may not accurately reflect the actual numbers of cases of AIDS. Thus, only 5,130 cases had been reported to WHO by 31 African countries by August 1987, though their actual number can be estimated to be at least tens of thousands . . .
> The annual incidence of AIDS in Kinshasa, Zaire, was estimated at 550–1000 cases per million people in 1984–1985 . . .[62]

We discussed these "back of the envelope" statistics earlier in the book (see page 40). Under their subsection titled "HIV seroprevalence", we read:

> Some initial serological surveys for HIV antibody in Africa yielded a high proportion of false positive reactions . . . Seroprevalence rates in healthy populations in Africa and the Caribbean vary widely. Results should always be interpreted with caution, since the way study subjects were selected may influence seroprevalence rates . . .[63]

Caution is then thrown to the winds, and we are served a variety of seroprevalence figures from old and recent studies of dubious scientific merit. The transmission of HIV infection by blood transfusions within Africa is discussed, but there is not a whisper of the use of imported blood products from Europe and America, although the authors must know that the practice was widespread before screening for HIV was introduced in the West. Needless to say, both Peter Piot and Anthony Pinching are on the Panos Institute's "expert advisory panel".[64]

Unsolved problems of seroepidemiology

Although there now seems to be general agreement that the early seroepidemiology studies in Africa were unreliable, AIDS researchers would like us to believe that these problems have been solved with the development of a new generation of ELISA tests. This optimism would seem unfounded, as false positivity remains a problem even in the West. The problem was discussed in a paper published in the *New England Journal of Medicine*, titled "Screening for HIV: Can we afford the false positive rate?":

> The central issue is the false positive rate of tests for HIV infection. Current screening programs use a sequence of tests, starting with an enzyme immunoassay [ELISA]. Serum samples yielding repeatedly positive results on enzyme immunoassay are subjected to more complicated and expensive confirmatory testing, typically with a Western blot. A positive confirmatory test is considered evidence of HIV infection . . .
>
> The Western blot . . . is complex and very labour intensive. Its techniques have not been standardised, and the magnitude and consequences of interlaboratory variations have not been measured. Its results require interpretation, and the criteria for this interpretation vary not only from laboratory to laboratory but also from month to month.[65]

The false positive rate for the ELISA test varied from zero to 0.42% when used for screening blood donors, but was as high as 6.8% among hospitalised patients. A confirmatory test such as the Western blot reduces the false positive rate. However, as the authors explain, unless the false positive rate for Western blot can be established, the joint false positive rate for the two tests cannot be determined. The authors then considered the implications of screening 100,000 people with a disease prevalence of 0.01% with tests with a joint false positive rate of 0.005%. If the tests were 100% sensitive, all 10 infected people would be correctly identified, but in addition there would be 5 positive results from people who were not infected. If the joint false positive rate was 0.5%, then 50 people without HIV infection would yield positive results for each truly infected person.

As the incidence of HIV infection in the population increases, the proportion of false positives detected will decline. However, it would seem that no conclusions about the incidence of HIV infection in a population can be reached unless the false positive rate is known with some reliability, and this will vary with the population tested, eg hospitalised patients, patients with a high incidence of chronic malaria, and so on. Western AIDS researchers discussing the AIDS situation in Africa, though, are not prone to self-doubt:

> Initial sero-epidemiological surveys in Kenya and Uganda reported prevalence data as high as 79% in rural people. However, these were almost entirely false-positive results caused by nonspecifically "sticky" antibodies (usually IgM) often found in the blood of Africans, possibly as a result of repeated parasitic infections . . .
>
> Nevertheless, subsequent studies using more specific tests for HIV antibodies (enzyme-linked immunosorbent assays – ELISA) have indeed revealed a major epidemic . . . A survey carried out in 1984 among 2384 hospital employees in Kinshasa, Zaire gave a prevalence of 6% with a rate of seroconversion of about 1% per annum . . .[66]

If new-generation ELISAs still yield a false positive rate of 6.8% in hospitalised patients in the West, can they really be reliable in apparently healthy subjects with chronic malaria and other parasitic diseases in Africa? The findings of a very large seroepidemiological study in six countries of central Africa were presented at the 1988 Stockholm conference. The seroprevalence rates in the general population varied from 0 to 7.5% and were significantly higher in adults and in urban areas, with females more commonly affected than males. The conclusions of the study were summarised as follows:

> Sera Elisa+/WB– are numerous and the Western Blotting tests show non-specific bands. The problem of the interpretation of these sera is still unsolved.[67]

The real situation in Africa

A London-based Ghanaian physician, Dr Konotey-Ahulu, became concerned about the reports of African AIDS in the medical literature and the popular press. He toured all the supposedly AIDS-affected African countries (except Zaire, where he was refused entry) to assess the situation. He reported his findings in *The Lancet*:

> In February and March of this year [1987] I made a six-week tour of twenty-six cities and towns in sixteen sub-Saharan countries, including those most afflicted by AIDS, did ward rounds with doctors and nurses, met ministers of health, directors of medical services, and research workers (native and expatriate) . . .
>
> If one judges the extent of AIDS in Africa on an arbitrary scale from grade I (not much of a problem) to grade V (a catastrophe), in my assessment AIDS is a problem (grade II) in only five (possibly six, since I was unable to obtain a visa for Zaire) of the countries where AIDS has

occurred . . . In no country is the AIDS problem consistently grade III (a great problem), or ever grade IV (an extremely great problem), and in none can it be called a catastrophe (grade V). In Kenya, for instance, contrary to widespread reports, I would rate AIDS in 1987 as grade I . . .

Before the days of AIDS in Ghana there was a death a day . . . on my ward alone of thirty-four beds . . . They died from one or another of the following: cerebrovascular accident from malignant hypertension, hepatoma, ruptured amoebic abscess, haematemesis, chronic renal failure, sickle-cell crisis, septicaemia, perforated typhoid gut, hepatic coma, haemoptysis from tuberculosis, brain tumour, Hodgkin's disease . . . Today, because of AIDS, it seems that Africans are not allowed to die from these conditions any longer. If tens of thousands are dying from AIDS (and Africans do not cremate their dead) where are the graves? . . .

"Why do the world's media appear to have conspired with some scientists to become so gratuitously extravagant with the untruth?" – that was the question uppermost in the minds of intelligent Africans and Europeans I met on my tour.[68]

In another article published in the *British Medical Journal*, Dr Konotey-Ahulu discussed the problems of seroepidemiology:

If there is one thing veteran physicians, surgeons, public health experts, and other health workers in Africa have been good at, it is clinical epidemiology. The work of Dr Cicely Williams (on kwashiorkor in West Africa) and Dr Denis Burkitt (on lymphoma in East Africa) is a prime example of what careful clinical and epidemiological observation can produce . . .

Now, suddenly, with the acquired immune deficiency syndrome (AIDS), something called seroepidemiology is being pushed – by people who have no knowledge of tropical medicine – way above clinical epidemiology, rather than being made to work shoulder to shoulder with it. While travelling extensively in sub-Saharan Africa I encountered grave disquiet about this approach. For example, Dr Miriam Duggan, the obstetrician-gynecologist medical superintendent of the large St Francis Hospital Nsabya, in Kampala, was saddened by the way that external research agencies lost interest whenever she mentioned the need for strengthening her clinical epidemiological research base to enable her to go around the villages to follow up and treat patients with AIDS who had been discharged, and to measure longevity. Research funds must never be for service . . ., she seems to have been told, but are for taking blood from as many people as possible to measure "seropositivity" and T lymphocytes . . .

During my travels through sub-Saharan Africa I was heartened to observe that there are enough trained health workers in post who can work out the clinical epidemiology of AIDS à la Cicely Williams and Burkitt with a minimum of fuss . . . Primary health care in Ghana, for instance, is so good that there is no difficulty in tracing patients with AIDS and their relatives . . .[69]

Although clinical epidemiology will give a far more accurate picture of the incidence of AIDS than seroepidemiological studies, there is accumulating evidence that clinical criteria used without reliable confirmatory testing will also produce a substantial overestimate of the scale of the problem. A study was undertaken at the Mama Yemo Hospital in Kinshasa, Zaire, to evaluate the WHO clinical case definition of AIDS.[70] Altogether 190 patients were classified according to the WHO criteria and tested for AIDS antibodies with ELISA, confirmed with either Western blot or indirect immuno-fluorescence; ie if one confirmatory test was negative, the sample was tested with the other. This is a strange procedure, as a negative result on one test would arouse suspicions of a false positive result on the other, but we are not told how many were positive with one test and not the other. The study showed that the positive predictive value of the WHO criteria was 74%; ie 26% of patients with clinical manifestations of AIDS were not seropositive. In the study by De Cock, Piot et al in Equater province, Zaire, 31 patients in local hospitals were found to have at least one of the features of AIDS described in the WHO clinical case definition, and 10 met the criteria for a diagnosis of AIDS.[71] Only 5 of these 10 patients were antibody positive. Studies in Uganda have shown that between 50 and 65% of patients who fulfilled the clinical criteria were seronegative (see page 107).

Even patients who were true seropositives are not necessarily AIDS cases (ie patients with opportunistic infections or tumours), as the WHO clinical criteria will also identify patients who have AIDS-related complex, the pre-AIDS syndrome that is considerably more common than AIDS itself. In the West, only cases of full-blown AIDS are reported, and African countries defining cases according to WHO criteria will still overestimate the incidence of AIDS even when using confirmatory tests. Western AIDS researchers frequently assert that there are many undiagnosed AIDS cases in Africa. However, as Dr Konotey-Ahulu has pointed out, it would be relatively easy for researchers to find AIDS cases, if they really did exist in large numbers.

Doctors in Uganda have been investigating the diagnostic dilemmas posed by AIDS, and a senior lecturer at Makerere University Medical School presented a paper at the 1988 Stockholm AIDS conference titled "The clinical manifestations of AIDS in an African population – some diagnostic pitfalls":

> In most developing African countries, the diagnosis of AIDS depends on the WHO clinical case definition. Unfortunately, confirmatory tests are rarely available, and in an analysis of over 500 patients who fulfilled the

WHO clinical case definition but were HIV-serology negative, various conditions were identified as potential diagnostic pitfalls.

Infections, particularly tuberculosis, other bacterial infections, hidden pus and parasitic infestations very often mimic AIDS. Lymphomas and occult carcinomas often present with prolonged fever and cachexia akin to "SLIM" disease. Endocrine disorders, such as diabetes mellitus, thyrotoxicosis and Addison's disease, cause weight loss and dermato-mucosal features similar to those of AIDS.

Other misleading conditions include mosquito bites, scabies and skin drug reactions. Some individuals who develop extreme fear of AIDS present with anxiety and somatic features such as diarrhoea, anorexia, weight loss, fatigue and night sweats leading to a mistaken diagnosis of the disease.[72]

It is interesting to note that AIDS researchers were not the first to predict the demise of the Ugandan population. In 1908 *The Lancet* commented on a report from Colonel FJ Lambkin, of the Royal Army Medical Corps:

> As things are at present the entire population [of Uganda] is in danger of being exterminated by Syphilis in a very few years, or of being left a degenerate race fit for nothing.[73]

Perhaps they have got it wrong again.

African Ministries of Health are now taking a closer look at their reported AIDS cases. In the WHO Weekly Epidemiological Record published in May 1988, Zimbabwe officially retracted the report of 380 cases pending a national review of the accuracy of the reporting system,[74] and subsequently reported a revised figure of 119 cases up to April 30 1988.[75] Two thirds of the previously reported cases, on closer investigation, were not found to be cases of AIDS. Zimbabwe has introduced wide-scale confirmatory testing with Western blot and has facilities for virus isolation. Blood samples are also sent abroad for further tests. The WHO Weekly Epidemiological Record in August 1988 also reported that the Gambia had revised its figures from 35 to 9 cases,[76] and in October 1988 the Sudan revised its figures from 82 to 68 cases.[77] One is left to wonder about the true incidence of AIDS in the east and central African states that have reported the greatest number of cases.

The new panic: the heterosexual spread from Africa

Although the supposed African origin of AIDS is receiving less emphasis in the medical literature, Africans are increasingly being perceived as responsible for the heterosexual spread of AIDS in Europe. For example, in March 1987 *The Lancet* published a paper titled "Acquired immunodeficiency syndrome after travelling in Africa: an epidemiological study in seventeen Caucasian patients" by a group of 13 French doctors from 9 hospitals, including the Pasteur Institute:

> Seventeen Caucasian patients with acquired immunodeficiency syndrome (AIDS) contracted after long stays in Africa are reported . . . This study suggests that the risk of contracting AIDS in Africa is high; the transmission of the virus was related to sexual contact, particularly with prostitutes, in Africa in most cases. It suggests that Caucasians who travel in Africa spread the virus throughout the world by means of their heterosexual relations.[78]

The French had reported 1,221 cases of AIDS to the WHO by December 1986,[79] at the time this paper was accepted for publication. The contribution of 17 cases acquired heterosexually in Africa to the French epidemic would be negligible, but even some of these are questionable. Two patients, admitted to hospital in 1976 and 1978, were diagnosed retrospectively "since a diagnosis of AIDS is very likely". One was married to a Zairean man who is alive and healthy more than ten years later, and who has not been tested for HIV. The other had lived in Mozambique from 1968 to 1976, and we are told that he had occasional sexual relations with prostitutes in Africa. One wonders whether the clinical history as well as the diagnosis were obtained posthumously; or perhaps the French doctors routinely ask their patients for details about their sex lives and carefully record the answers in the case notes. AIDS in Mozambique has appeared only very recently, and it is curious that an expatriate would acquire a disease a decade before the epidemic appeared in the local population. A third case was a child born in Africa to a Zairean father and a French mother. The child was seronegative on three tests – ELISA, radioimmunoprecipitation assay and Western blot. We should remind ourselves of the title of the paper, "Acquired immunodeficiency syndrome after travelling in Africa: an epidemiological study in seventeen Caucasian patients", yet here is a patient who was neither Caucasian, travelling in Africa, nor even seropositive for HIV. Moreover, one patient was a bisexual who had regular homosexual relations with one healthy African partner. Two thirds of the 1,221 French cases reported by December 1986 were homosexuals, and only one apparently caught the infection in Africa. Are the authors of this paper seriously suggesting that African heterosexuals are significantly influencing the epidemic amongst French homosexuals?

Another patient, a young female student, had a blood transfusion in the Cameroons 16 months before she developed AIDS in May

1985. Some of the poorer African countries, like the Cameroons, do not have the resources to maintain a blood transfusion service and import blood from Europe or America or arrange for an immediate transfusion from a relative or friend. It is most unlikely that a French woman would have received a transfusion from a local Cameroonian and quite possible that she was transfused with imported blood. Routine screening of blood products began in the West in 1984 and, according to a WHO working paper, unscreened blood products may have been dumped on Third World countries:

> Due to poor socio-economic conditions in many developing countries, it is not possible to organise efficient blood transfusion services quickly. The situation was immediately used by the commercial plasma industry, which made good profit from the trade in blood . . .
> At the beginning of the AIDS crisis it was said that products from contaminated plasma pools were sold at discount prices in developing countries since they could not check the products. Legal proceedings against some companies said to have supplied the infected plasma have been started.[80]

If we discount these 5 cases from the original 17, we are left with 12 heterosexual men who developed AIDS between 1984 and 1986. One sick man was unable to give a history, but the remaining 11 had sexual relations with prostitutes in Africa, 5 occasionally and 6 frequently. All of these men had also had sexual relations outside Africa, mostly in France, but we are not told whether with prostitutes or not. If these men did have sexual relations with prostitutes in France and in Africa, why should we assume that they were infected in Africa? Many European prostitutes are also intravenous drug abusers, and the seropositivity rate is comparable with or even higher than seropositivity in African prostitutes (see pages 105 and 106).
Like so many AIDS researchers, the authors assume that HIV can be transmitted only from Africans to Europeans, and never the reverse; they do not even consider the possibility that Frenchmen could have spread AIDS to Africa, even though France has the second highest number of AIDS cases in the world, after the United States. Towards the end of the paper the French researchers state:

> Our study confirms that prostitutes constitute a reservoir of HIV, particularly in central Africa, and suggests that the virus will continue to spread through heterosexual contacts . . . The best way to estimate the risk of HIV infection would be to evaluate the probability of becoming seropositive in unmarried Caucasian men living in Africa, such as soldiers, a year after arrival in the continent.[81]

A group of Belgian researchers took this advice, and published their findings in a leading article in the *British Medical Journal*:

The pattern of cases of AIDS in Belgium suggests that Europeans infected with human immunodeficiency virus (HIV) acquired the infection in Africa . . . Fifteen (1.1%) of 1,401 Belgian advisers working in Africa and 41 (0.9%) of 4,564 European expatriates living in Africa were positive for antibody to HIV in a voluntary screening programme in Belgium . . .[82]

The study was confined to men, as they detected only 14 women who had antibody to HIV, half of whom had had sexual relations with one seropositive man whose nationality was not stated. The participants were asked to complete a self-administered questionnaire, which included questions on sociodemographic characteristics and risk factors for infection with HIV. American studies have shown that self-administered questionnaires are less likely to reveal risk factors than personal interviews:

Another approach to monitoring for heterosexually acquired infection is measuring the HIV antibody prevalence among patients in STD [sexually transmitted disease] clinics who, through interview, are carefully determined not to have recognized sexual, IV-drug-related, or blood- or blood-product-related risk factors . . . In nine surveys in six major cities, where HIV infection risk was evaluated rigorously through interview with the opportunity to reinterview seropositives, infection prevalence ranged from 0 to 1.2% among persons without identified risk factors. Where risk was evaluated less rigorously through an anonymous self-administered questionnaire, a prevalence as high as 2.6% was observed among persons not acknowledging risk.[83]

Perhaps Belgians are more honest than Americans, but the Belgian study was undertaken in the clinic of the Ministry of Foreign Affairs in Brussels and, although confidential, was not anonymous. An admission of homosexuality or intravenous drug abuse would be detrimental to a career in government service, whilst an admission of heterosexual promiscuity would not.

The HIV positive men, who had spent at least six months in sub-Saharan Africa during the previous five years, were compared with HIV negative men who had spent at least two years out of the previous five in sub-Saharan Africa. No explanation is offered for choosing different periods of residence in Africa for the two groups. Seropositivity was significantly associated with promiscuity, in particular sexual relations with prostitutes:

Men with antibody to HIV had had significantly more heterosexual partners, more African sexual partners, and more contact with prostitutes during the previous five years, and they also reported significantly more episodes of sexually transmitted diseases . . .

This prevalence is about 250 times higher than that among Belgian blood donors, of whom 0.004% had antibody to HIV in 1986 . . .

Sexual intercourse with local women, including a high proportion of prostitutes, was the most important risk factor for infection among expatriate men, with a strong relation between the number of such sexual partners and the odds of being infected with HIV. *Because of the prevalence of antibody to HIV (5% and higher) in some urban populations in central Africa, the likelihood of having sexual intercourse with an infected heterosexual partner is much higher than in Europe and North America. The risk is particularly high for intercourse with female prostitutes, of whom up to 88% are infected in central and eastern Africa.* [Our emphasis]

Our results show an additional route whereby HIV may be introduced into the heterosexual population in Europe and North America . . . The epidemiological data on AIDS in Belgium show that heterosexuals account for a significant proportion of cases in a European population and that secondary spread to the local population in Belgium is already occurring . . . Thus heterosexual transmission of HIV may become more common in continents other than Africa.[84]

Even if we assume that the seropositive men did not have other risk factors, how much credence can we give to these findings? There are a number of underlying assumptions in this study that the authors fail to question. We are told that the men were tested for HIV after they had been to Africa, but none, apparently, had been tested before he left. The incubation period from the time of infection to the development of symptoms for most sexually transmitted diseases is a matter of days, and the source of infection can usually be identified. With HIV infection it is many months or years, and the virus does not come with a tag saying "made in Brussels" or "made in Kinshasa". It is impossible to ascertain from the data presented whether the men were questioned only about their sexual activities in Africa or also about their previous activities in Europe. This is an important question: if the Belgians were more promiscuous in Africa, they could be at greater risk of acquiring HIV infection there, even if the rate of HIV infection was lower in Africa than in Belgium.

The authors claim that the risk of acquiring HIV infection is higher in Africa than in Europe because 5% of some urban populations in central Africa are infected with HIV. Even if these seroprevalence studies were believable, in this instance they are not particularly relevant. A high proportion of the women who supposedly infected the Belgians were prostitutes, and there is no consistent evidence that seropositivity is higher in African prostitutes than in their European counterparts. Although the authors mention one study that found a seroprevalence of 88%, a study in Kinshasa found 27% of prostitutes to be seropositive,[85] and rates in some European cities are comparable or higher (see page 106 of this book). The following testimony was presented to the US Congress back in 1985:

A recent survey completed in West Germany also indicates that the infection of the prostitute population is a problem of major proportions. Nationwide, about twenty percent of all prostitutes in Germany are infected . . . In one study, more than half of the unregistered prostitutes working in the area of Berlin near the train station were found to be infected.

There is accumulating evidence that infection is transmitted from prostitutes to their customers. A recent study conducted by the United States Army revealed that five percent of United States soldiers reporting to venereal disease clinics in Berlin are now infected with the AIDS virus . . . A lethal venereal disease is now spreading through our population, all the more dangerous because infections may remain inapparent for a long time.[86]

The situation in Glasgow was outlined in *New Scientist* in April 1988:

At least three-quarters of Glasgow's known female drug users infected with HIV are actively working as prostitutes to fund their drug habit. Moreover, many have sex with clients without the protection of a condom. Public education has clearly failed to diminish the demand for such services. Some prostitutes have up to 30 clients in a 24-hour period . . .

"The classic tale we hear is that men start out at the top of the hill in Glasgow – the 'better' area – where the prostitutes are not drug abusers, ask for sex without a condom, are refused and gradually work their way down the hill to where the infected drug misusers work. Invariably it's the drug misusers they end up with."[87]

European men who have unprotected sexual intercourse with prostitutes are at risk for HIV infection, whether they travel to Africa or stay at home.

The Belgians found that 1% of their expatriates were seropositive, and compared this with the low seropositivity of Belgian blood donors. Are such comparisons valid? Blood donors are a highly selected population with a low risk for HIV infection (although in neighbouring France the seropositivity of new blood donors was 1%, the same as the Belgians in this study).[88] The prevalence of HIV infection varies with age, sex, class, marital status, sexual orientation, promiscuity, etc. Men who had been to Africa can be compared with blood donors only if their stay in Africa was the only significant characteristic that distinguished the two groups. Although we have no information about the degree of promiscuity of the average Belgian man, about one third of the expatriate Belgians reported that they had sexual contact with prostitutes, and it seems very probable that Belgian men who go to Africa are a highly promiscuous, unrepresentative section of the Belgian population. Conclusions about the risks of a visit to Africa can be drawn only if the Belgians in

Africa were compared with a similarly promiscuous group who had either stayed in Belgium or travelled elsewhere. The possibility that promiscuous Belgian men may have infected Africans is not even considered, although AIDS appears to be particularly affecting prostitutes in Africa working in places frequented by foreign tourists.[89] It is quite extraordinary that these researchers can perceive the widespread sexual exploitation of poor African women by their former colonial masters only as a threat posed by African sexuality to the health of Europe.

Political and military perspectives

Many Africans regard the AIDS epidemic in Africa as a deliberate attempt at mass extermination. If such views appear to be "over the top", it is salutary to read an article in the *International Defense Review* titled "AIDS: Its strategic consequences in black Africa". The article is illustrated by pictures of children in the age group least affected by AIDS, and of a freshly dug grave with a caption:

> Thousands of freshly dug graves like this litter the East African countryside, evidence of a massive catastrophe.[90]

The contents of the article are even more disturbing. There are the usual accounts of truck drivers spreading AIDS, African green monkeys as the source of the epidemic and the various ways they may have transmitted AIDS to humans, such as the use of monkey blood as a sexual stimulant. Although we are told that the World Health Organisation estimated there were 2 million African AIDS cases, the author of the article had to admit that there was little evidence of the disease visible in everyday life in the cities he visited, with the exception of a shortage of prostitutes hanging around hotels in Kampala. According to the article the United States has recently established its own AIDS research unit in the Kenyan capital, under the command of General Phillip K. Russell. The unit reports back directly to the US Army virus research authority at Fort Detrick, at Frederick, Maryland, and is headed by Dr Bruce Johnson, who has been in Kenya for several years.

Why the American military should be so interested in the African AIDS situation becomes clear later in the article. Dr Johnson himself refused to be interviewed, but we are told that he was seeing 25 cases of suspected AIDS each day. This same Dr Johnson also claimed that sexually transmitted AIDS appeared in children of about 12 to 13 years of age, "when many black children become sexually active". No substantiation is provided for this ridiculous assertion. Of course African governments are accused of a "conspiracy of silence";

supposedly 50% of the Zambian armed forces are infected (they surely cannot pose much of a military threat), Eastern European diplomatic personnel have become infected and are now sent home if they consort with local girls, and the rest are being tested every six months. Apparently even African National Congress guerillas and several members of the ANC command structure have come down with AIDS, and so on.

The most interesting section of the article, though, deals with the strategic implications:

> The potential depopulation of much of Black Africa holds serious consequences for the international community. Africa is still the world's largest single commodities resource, from uranium, copper and gold all the way through to hundreds of consumer items as diverse as cocoa, hardwoods, maize and a host of tropical products . . .
>
> But what if current projections are correct, and more than half the population of countries like Uganda, Kenya, Zaire and much of equatorial West Africa are wiped out before the turn of the century?
>
> Who will fill the vacuum? Immense tracts of African real estate will become available, literally for the taking, because national forces will be unable to do anything about it.
>
> Clearly, this is one of the issues being carefully assessed by the United States with its Department of Defense presence in Nairobi. If there is any major step to be taken, the Americans want to be the first to implement it.
>
> A curious sidelight in East Africa is the attitude of the local Asian and European residents. Some whites in Nairobi refer rather cynically to Kenya as a good place to buy property for the future. It could well be one reason why property prices in Kenya have risen rather sharply of late.
>
> But it is the Asian community which takes a rather more serious view of the matter. Some Asians in Nairobi are already talking of a depopulated East Africa being ideal for the settlement of some of continental India's overpopulation. Indian communities have been in Africa for more than a century and have proved themselves highly adaptable.
>
> It could be that a major Indian migration would turn Africa into the continent of the future. With the economic gusto and enterprise which Indians have shown in dozens of countries around the globe, they could be the best influence Africa has seen for generations. Certainly, they could change the economic face of a continent at present slipping into somnolent chaos.
>
> For their part, the South Africans would react strongly. If Zambia or Mozambique were depopulated, South Africa would surely try to fill that gap with its own forces. There are some strategists in Pretoria already talking about a new "buffer concept", several hundred kilometers north of the existing borders . . .
>
> Certainly Africa, with its extensive reserves of strategic ores and minerals, will be much in the limelight in the decades ahead. Should Zambia, with its copper, or Zaire, with its cobalt, copper, diamonds, gold

and uranium, go to waste as a consequence of AIDS, it will be interesting to see at what stage the developed world starts its new scramble for Africa.[91]

The most frightening thing about this article is not that it may be true (it is nonsense) but that powerful interest groups in the West and South Africa wish it to be true. There is surely a contradiction between the ostensible humanitarian motives of the Western AIDS researchers in Africa and the underlying purposes of the Western governments providing them with the financial resources for their research. Such contradictions are not new, as any student of African history knows that Europeans colonised Africa with the Bible in one hand and the gun in the other.

Evidence for direct American government interest in the issue of AIDS in Africa appeared in the form of Kathleen Bailey, deputy assistant Secretary of State in the US Bureau of Intelligence and Research, who described her activities on behalf of the US government in an article in the *Los Angeles Times* (April 19 1987):

> In October 1985, the influential Soviet weekly *Literaturnaya Gazeta* published an article alleging that the US government had engineered the AIDS virus during biological warfare research . . .
> The disinformation was first planted in India because the most difficult obstacle the Soviets face in dealing with the Western press is that journalists insist on proper sources for a story . . .[92]

Such an assertion almost defies comment! "Proper sources" hardly describes the basis of articles about AIDS in Africa that have appeared in the Western popular and scientific press.

Ms Bailey then outlined the means by which the Soviet Union spread their supposed disinformation, and the harmful effects it could have on American interests:

> Some readers may ask what difference it makes. Does such a story really influence perceptions of the United States? Does it actually hurt US foreign policy? . . . A short answer can be provided by an anecdote.
> Because many scientists have speculated that the AIDS virus evolved in Africa and because the disease has taken its highest toll there, peoples on that continent are highly sensitive about the issue . . .[93]

How can an American government official claim to be countering disinformation whilst denying that the great majority of AIDS cases were occurring in the United States? When Ms Bailey was touring Africa, the United States had reported 26,566 cases out of a world total of 34,448, whilst only 1,069 cases had been reported from the whole of Africa.[94] She appreciated that Africans were none too keen to claim responsibility for AIDS:

Knowing that many Africans might unconsciously welcome an alternative explanation for AIDS' origin, the Soviets focused much of the disinformation campaign on African media . . . Because this campaign – as well as other disinformation efforts – were so active in Africa, I visited there in November 1986.

One evening, an African government official was telling me about the severity of the AIDS epidemic in his country. He began to chastise me for the United States having created the virus. I asked him why he thought so and he responded, "Obviously the United States is technically capable of almost anything. Also, why should such a story be in so many newspapers if it were not true?"

Only after detailing for him the origin of the story and providing statements from leading scientists, including Soviets, on the impossibility of artificially creating the virus, did he change his view.[95]

Unfortunately for the American government, the possibility of a laboratory origin cannot be dismissed so easily. Now that researchers have failed to find their lost tribes who had supposedly harboured HIV for centuries, and African green monkeys have been absolved from responsibility, there is accumulating evidence that the human immunodeficiency virus is most closely related to sheep and cattle viruses that cause wasting diseases similar to AIDS.[96,97] Visna, the sheep virus, was successfully grown in human cell culture in 1962[98] and has been the subject of a series of experiments, some of which were undertaken by scientists, including Gallo and Essex, who are now AIDS experts.[99] Laboratory animals, including sub-human primates, have been experimentally infected with these viruses. It is little wonder that both Kathleen Bailey and many of these scientists are so ready to blame Africa.

There may also be very direct, practical reasons to portray Africa as the epicentre of the world's AIDS epidemic. The subject of vaccine trials was discussed by Silvia Federici in an article titled "White doctors in Africa (on the trail of AIDS, or in service of the empire?)":

For those like myself who grew up in the immediate aftermath of World War II, the thought of experiments on humans always evokes images of Nazi concentration camps. So when Dr Anthony Fauci, director of the National Institute of Allergy and Infectious Diseases, announced that the United States is planning to conduct large scale human experiments in Africa to test potential AIDS vaccines (*New York Times*, Feb. 19 1988), I would have expected – if not a public outcry – at least some questions of the type our media are quick to bring up when discussing, say, "human rights abuses" by the Sandinistas.

Consider, we have repeatedly been told that there is *no* safe method, at present, for conducting such tests on humans, since even in the presence of antibodies it is possible to contract AIDS. And of course that's why very few people here in the US (54, to be precise) will be tested upon – and why, in their case, we are given ample assurance that no part of the HIV virus will be used (*New York Times*, August 26 1988) . . .

Why then so much indifference towards the well-being of Africans? One possible reason is that public conscience has been appeased by the official explanation, which tells us that Africa provides a "natural" lab because AIDS in Africa is supposedly "spreading like wildfire". From this we are expected to deduce that the tests are in line with the best utilitarian tradition, that times of extreme hardship demand the sacrifice of a few for the benefit of the majority.

However, *no* reliable evidence has so far been presented to support these claims of an African AIDS pandemic . . . the real secret behind the choice of Africa is the assumed cheapness of African lives . . .

Unfortunately, it's all too true that, for the sake of a little hard currency, *some* African governments can be blackmailed into delivering their citizens over to unscrutinized medical experimentation, in the same way that some are now turning their countries into dumping grounds for chemical and radioactive waste, in exchange for dollars or pounds . . .

That this is no idle fear is taught by our own past experience. A case in point is the infamous Tuskegee study, when the Centers for Disease Control deliberately withheld treatment for decades from Southern black sharecroppers, in order to "follow the development" of syphilis through all its stages, even unto the grave.

If this sort of atrocity could continue in the United States as late as 1972, when the "study" ceased only because it was finally exposed, just imagine what can happen in countries like Zaire – countries the US controls politically, whose economies are at the mercy of the International Monetary Fund, and where abuses of human rights are the order of the day?[100]

Perhaps Africans should be seeking the support of the Animal Liberation Front! Certainly we shall not be safe if left to the tender mercies of the AIDS researchers.

The acquired immune deficiency syndrome is undoubtedly the most political disease of modern times, and the direction and purpose of so much AIDS research cannot be understood unless this political dimension is appreciated. Why, for example, was it necessary for Reagan and Chirac to meet at the White House to agree on an official history of the discovery of AIDS? As the possibility of the accidental production of a lethal virus was considered and debated by the scientists themselves as early as 1966,[101] why has the scientific community, with few exceptions, been unwilling to consider a laboratory origin for the AIDS virus? Why have the scientists been so determined to associate Africa with the source and dissemination of AIDS when the most basic epidemiological evidence points to the United States? Furthermore, Peter Piot and Joseph McCormick worked closely with the American and South African military in

Zaire in the 1970s. How many more of the scientists who now dominate AIDS research have had previous links with secret military research establishments?

We have shown how racism has guided the direction of AIDS research; moreover, that the problem is not simply the subjective prejudices of individual AIDS researchers but a racist world-view that coincides with the material self-interest of research institutions and of the Western governments that fund them. There is an illusion that science is objective, that scientists search for the truth irrespective of outside pressures. In reality the only science that exists is the science that is done, and he who pays the piper calls the tune.

References
1. New Scientist. *Evidence for origin is weak*. October 15, 1987, p27.
2. *HIV origin "a continuing mystery": green monkey theory disputed*. Skin and Allergy News, January 1988, p28.
3. C Mulder. *A case of mistaken non-identity*. Nature, Vol 331, February 18, 1988, p562–3.
4. HW Kestler, Y Li et al. *Comparison of simian immunodeficiency virus isolates*, Nature, Vol 331, February 18, 1988, p619–21.
5. M Essex, P Kanki. *Reply to Kestler et al*. Nature, Vol 331, February 18, 1988, p621–2.
6. *Laboratory mix-up solves AIDS mystery*. New Scientist, February 25, 1988, p32.
7. C Mulder. *Human virus not from monkeys*. Nature, Vol 333, June 2, 1988, p396.
8. MA Gonda, F Wong-Staal, RC Gallo et al. *Sequence homology and morphologic similarity of HTLV-III and Visna virus, a pathogenic lentivirus*. Science, Vol 227, January 11, 1985, p173–7.
9. MA Gonda, MJ Braun, SG Carter et al. *Characterization and molecular cloning of a bovine lentivirus related to human immunodeficiency virus*. Nature, Vol 330, No 6146, p388–91, November 26, 1987.
10. J Grote. *Bovine visna virus and the origin of HIV*. Journal of the Royal Society of Medicine, Vol 81, October 1988, p620.
11. J Seale. *Origins of the AIDS viruses, HIV-1 and HIV-2: fact or fiction? Discussion paper*. Journal of the Royal Society of Medicine, Vol 81, September 1988, p537–9.
12. P Nunn, KPWJ McAdam. *AIDS in Africa*. Medicine International, September 1988, p2357–60.
13. AJ Pinching, RA Weiss, D Miller. *AIDS and HIV infection: new perspectives*. British Medical Bulletin, Vol 44, No 1, January 1988, p4.
14. P Tauris, FT Black. *Heterosexuals importing HIV from Africa*. The Lancet, February 7, 1987, p325.
15. D Vittecoq, RT Roue, C Mayaud et al. *Acquired immunodeficiency*

syndrome after travelling in Africa: an epidemiological study in seventeen Caucasian patients. The Lancet, March 14, 1987, p612–4.

16. L Bonneux, P Van der Stuyft, H Taelman et al. *Risk factors for infection with human immunodeficiency virus among European expatriates in Africa.* British Medical Journal, Vol 297, September 3, 1988, p581–4.

17. op cit C Mulder. *A case of mistaken non-identity.*

18. op cit HW Kestler, Y Li et al.

19. op cit M Essex, P Kanki. *Reply to Kestler et al.*

20. op cit *Laboratory mix-up solves AIDS mystery.*

21. op cit C Mulder. *Human virus not from monkeys.*

22. R Sabatier. *Don't blame Africa yet.* The Guardian, March 8, 1988.

23. M Fukasawa, T Miura, A Hasegawa et al. *Sequence of simian immunodeficiency virus from African green monkey, a new member of the HIV/SIV group.* Nature, Vol 333, June 2, 1988, p457–60.

24. op cit C Mulder. *Human AIDS virus not from monkeys.*

25. M Essex, P Kanki. *The origins of the AIDS virus.* Scientific American, October 1988, p44–51.

26. HP Katner, GA Pankey. *Evidence for a Euro-American origin of human immunodeficiency virus.* Journal National Medical Association, Vol 79, 1987, p1068–72.

27. op cit J Seale.

28. J Segal, L Segal. *AIDS – Natur und Ursprung. In AIDS Erreger aus dem Genlabor?* K Kruse ed. Simon and Leutner, Berlin 1987, p78–127.

29. op cit MA Gonda, F Wong-Staal, RC Gallo et al.

30. op cit MA Gonda, MJ Braun, SG Carter et al.

31. op cit J Grote.

32. F Clavel, D Guetard, F Brun-Vezinet et al. *Isolation of a new human retrovirus from West African patients with AIDS.* Science, Vol 233, July 18, 1986, p343–6.

33. *Acquired immunodeficiency syndrome (AIDS) – data as at 30 September 1988.* Weekly Epidemiological Record No 41, October 7, 1988, p309–10.

34. FID Konotey-Ahulu. *AIDS in Africa: Misinformation and disinformation.* The Lancet, July 25, 1987, p206–8.

35. op cit R Sabatier. *The Guardian,* March 8, 1988.

36. *New technique reveals extent of viral variations.* New Scientist, June 23, 1988, p37.

37. N Nzilambi, K De Cock, DN Forthal et al. *The prevalence of infection with human immunodeficiency virus over a 10-year period in rural Zaire.* The New England Journal of Medicine, February 4, 1988, p276–9.

38. B Davidson. *Africa in History.* Granada Publishing Limited, 1978, p150–153.

39. JP Getchell, DR Hicks, A Svinivasan et al. *Human immunodeficiency virus isolated from a serum sample collected in 1976 in central Africa.* The Journal of Infectious Diseases, Vol 156, No 5, November 1987, p833–7.

40. RF Garry, MH Witte, AA Gottlieb et al. *Documentation of an AIDS*

virus infection in the United States in 1968. Journal of the American Medical Association, Vol 260, 1988, p2085–7.

41. RJ Biggar, PC Nasca, WS Burnett. *AIDS-related Kaposi's sarcoma in New York City in 1977.* The New England Journal of Medicine, January 28, 1988, p252.
42. op cit *New Scientist*, October 15, 1987, p27.
43. IC Bygbjerg. *AIDS in a Danish surgeon (Zaire, 1976).* The Lancet, April 23, 1983, p925.
44. R Shilts. *And the Band Played On.* St Martin's Press, New York, pxiv.
45. Letter from Dr Bygbjerg to Dr Grote, April 18, 1988.
46. Personal communication.
47. Poster presentation at AIDS and Africa conference, Naples, October 1987.
48. op cit HP Katner, GA Pankey.
49. ibid HP Katner, GA Pankey.
50. op cit *New Scientist*, October 15, 1987, p27.
51. op cit *Skin and Allergy News*, January 1988.
52. F Noireau. *HIV transmission from monkey to man.* The Lancet, June 27, 1987, p1498–9.
53. op cit *Skin and Allergy News*, January 1988.
54. op cit P Nunn, PWJ McAdam. *Medicine International.*
55. ibid P Nunn, PWJ McAdam.
56. R Sabatier. *Blaming Others.* The Panos Institute, 1988, p166.
57. op cit P Nunn, PWJ McAdam pU240.
58. *Searchlight*, July 1988.
59. AJ Pinching, RA Weiss, D Miller. *AIDS and HIV infection: the wider perspective.* British Medical Bulletin, Vol 44, No 1, 1988, p4.
60. FID Konotey-Ahulu. *Group specific component and HIV infection.* The Lancet, May 30, 1987, p1267.
61. AR Moss. *Epidemiology of AIDS in developed countries.* British Medical Bulletin, Vol 44, No 1, 1988, p58.
62. P Piot, M Carael. *Epidemiological and sociological aspects of HIV-infection in developing countries.* British Medical Bulletin, Vol 44, No 1, 1988, p69.
63. ibid P Piot, M Carael p70.
64. op cit R Sabatier. *Blaming Others.*
65. KB Meyer, SG Pauker. *Screening for HIV: Can we afford the false positive rate?* The New England Journal of Medicine, Vol 317, No 4, July 23, 1987, p238–41.
66. op cit P Nunn, PWJ McAdam p2357.
67. R Josse, E Delaporte, L Kaptue et al. *Continuing studies on seroepidemiological surveys of HIV infection in central Africa: About 35 sample surveys.* Presented at the 4th International Conference on AIDS, Stockholm 1988.
68. FID Konotey-Ahulu. *AIDS in Africa: Misinformation and Disinformation.* The Lancet, July 25, 1987, p206–7.
69. FID Konotey-Ahulu. *Clinical epidemiology, not seroepidemiology, is the answer to Africa's AIDS problem.* British Medical Journal, Vol 294,

20 June, 1987, p1593–4.

70. R Colebunders, H Francis, L Izaley et al. *Evaluation of a clinical case definition of acquired immunodeficiency syndrome in Africa.* The Lancet, February 28, 1987, p492–4.

71. op cit N Nzilambi, K De Cock, DN Forthal et al.

72. RD Mugerwa. *The clinical manifestations of AIDS in an African population – some diagnostic pitfalls.* Presented at the 4th International Conference on AIDS, Stockholm 1988.

73. *Syphilis in Uganda.* The Lancet, October 3, 1908, p1022–3.

74. *Acquired Immunodeficiency Syndrome (AIDS) – Data as at 30 April 1988.* WHO Weekly Epidemiological Record No 19, May 6, 1988, p138–9.

75. *Acquired Immunodeficiency Syndrome (AIDS) – Data as at 31 July 1988.* WHO Weekly Epidemiological Record No 32, August 5, 1988, p241–2.

76. ibid WHO Weekly Epidemiological Record No 32, August 5, 1988, p241–2.

77. *Acquired Immunodeficiency Syndrome (AIDS) – Data as at 30 September 1988.* WHO Weekly Epidemiological Record No 41, October 7, 1988, p309–10.

78. op cit D Vittecoq, RT Roue, C Mayaud et al.

79. *Acquired immunodeficiency syndrome (AIDS): Situation in the WHO European region as of 31 December 1986.* WHO Weekly Epidemiological Record No 17, April 24, 1987, p117–21.

80. B Bytchenko. *The role of quality control of blood and blood products in AIDS containment.* WHO – "Working Papers" AIDS-Forschung (AIFO), September 1986, Heft 9, p495–6.

81. op cit D Vittecoq, RT Roue, C Mayaud et al.

82. op cit L Bonneux, P Van der Stuyft, H Taelman et al.

83. *Human immunodeficiency virus infection in the United States: a review of current knowledge.* Morbidity and Mortality Weekly Report, Vol 36, No 5–6, December 18, 1987, p1–21.

84. op cit L Bonneux, P Van der Stuyft, H Taelman et al.

85. op cit N Nzilambi, K De Cock, DN Forthal et al.

86. WA Haseltine. *HTLV-III/LAV-antibody-positive soldiers in Berlin.* The Lancet, Vol 314, No 1, January 2, 1986, p55–6.

87. *Infected prostitutes continue to work.* New Scientist, April 14, 1988.

88. *Acquired immunodeficiency syndrome (AIDS): HIV antibody screening in blood transfusion establishments.* WHO Weekly Epidemiological Record No 40, September 30, 1988, p302–4.

89. FID Konotey-Ahulu. *AIDS: origin, transmission and moral dilemmas.* Journal of the Royal Society of Medicine, Vol 80, November 1987, p720.

90. AJ Venter. *AIDS: Its strategic consequences in Black Africa.* International Defense Review 4/1988.

91. ibid AJ Venter.

92. K Bailey. *Soviets sponsor spread of AIDS disinformation.* Los Angeles Times, April 19, 1986.

93. ibid K Bailey.
94. *Acquired immunodeficiency syndrome (AIDS): Global data.* Weekly Epidemiological Record No 47, November 21, 1986, p361–3.
95. op cit K Bailey.
96. op cit MA Gonda, F Wong-Staal, RC Gallo et al.
97. op cit MA Gonda, MJ Braun, SG Carter et al.
98. H Thormar, B Sigurdardottir. *Growth of Visna virus in primary tissue cultures from various animals.* Acta Pathology and Microbiology of Scandinavia, Vol 55, 1962, p180–6.
99. See DR Strayer and DH Gillespie. *Virology monographs: The nature and organization of retroviral genes in animal cells.* Springer-Verlag, New York/Vienna.
100. S Federici. *White doctors in Africa (on the trail of AIDS, or in the service of the empire?).* Left Field, September 14, 1988.
101. FM Burnet. *Men or molecules? A tilt at molecular biology.* The Lancet, January 1, 1966, p37–9.

Appendix A

Provisional WHO clinical case definition for AIDS
(From the World Health Organisation's *Weekly Epidemiological Record* No 10, March 7, 1986, page 71.)

A *clinical* case definition is needed in countries where diagnostic resources are limited. A provisional clinical case definition was developed at a WHO Workshop on AIDS held in Bangui, Central African Republic, 22-24 October 1985. This definition was reviewed and slightly adapted at the Second Meeting of the WHO Collaborating Centres on AIDS as follows:

Adults

AIDS in an adult is defined by the existence of at least 2 of the major signs associated with at least 1 minor sign, in the absence of known causes of immunosuppression such as cancer or severe malnutrition or other recognized etiologies.

1. *Major signs*
   (a) weight loss $\geqslant$10% of body weight;
   (b) chronic diarrhoea >1 month;
   (c) prolonged fever >1 month (intermittent or constant).

2. *Minor signs*
   (a) persistent cough for >1 month;
   (b) generalized pruritic dermatitis;
   (c) recurrent herpes zoster;
   (d) oro-pharyngeal candidiasis;
   (e) chronic progressive and disseminated herpes simplex infection;
   (f) generalized lymphadenopathy.

The presence of generalized Kaposi's sarcoma or cryptococcal meningitis are sufficient by themselves for the diagnosis of AIDS.

Children

Paediatric AIDS is suspected in an infant or child presenting with at least 2 of the following major signs associated with at least 2 of the following minor signs in the absence of known causes of immunosuppression such as cancer or severe malnutrition or other recognized etiologies.

1. *Major signs*
   (a) weight loss or abnormally slow growth;
   (b) chronic diarrhoea >1 month;
   (c) prolonged fever >1 month.

2. *Minor signs*
   (a) generalized lymphadenopathy;
   (b) oro-pharyngeal candidiasis:
   (c) repeated common infections (otitis, pharyngitis, etc.);
   (d) persistent cough;
   (e) generalized dermatitis;
   (f) confirmed maternal LAV/HTLV-III infection.

Appendix B

Continental breakdown of AIDS cases reported to the World Health Organisation as of October 31, 1988

(Data from the WHO *Weekly Epidemiological Record* No 45, November 4, 1988, pp341–8.)

Africa

Country	Number of cases
Algeria	13
Angola	65
Benin	15
Botswana	34
Burkina Faso	26
Burundi	1,408
Cameroon	53
Cape Verde	4
Central African Republic	432
Chad	7
Comoros	1
Congo	1,250
Côte d'Ivoire	250
Djibouti	–
Egypt	6
Equatorial Guinea	–
Ethiopia	54
Gabon	18
Gambia*	52
Ghana	145
Guinea	10
Guinea Bissau	29
Kenya	2,732
Lesotho	2
Liberia	2
Libya	–
Madagascar	–
Malawi†	2,586
Mali	29
Mauritania	–

Mauritius	1
Morocco	12
Mozambique	10
Niger	9
Nigeria	11
Réunion	3
Rwanda	987
São Tomé and Principe	1
Senegal	131
Seychelles	–
Sierra Leone	5
Somalia	–
South Africa	135
Sudan	68
Swaziland	14
Togo	2
Tunisia	21
Uganda	4,006
United Republic of Tanzania	3,055
Zaire	335
Zambia	993
Zimbabwe	119
Total	**19,141**

The Americas

Country	Number of cases
Anguilla	1
Antigua and Barbuda	3
Argentina	197
Bahamas	214
Barbados	63
Belize	8
Bermuda	81
Bolivia	8
Brazil	3,687
British Virgin Islands	–
Canada	2,001
Cayman Islands	4
Chile	83

Colombia	244
Costa Rica	66
Cuba	34
Dominica	6
Dominican Republic	566
Ecuador	45
El Salvador	32
French Guiana	113
Grenada	11
Guadeloupe	74
Guatemala	39
Guyana	16
Haiti	1,455
Honduras	164
Jamaica	66
Martinique	38
Mexico	1,502
Monserrat	–
Nicaragua	1
Panama	64
Paraguay	8
Peru	98
Saint Christopher and Nevis	1
Saint Lucia	11
Saint Vincent and the Grenadines	10
Suriname	9
Trinidad and Tobago	302
Turks and Caicos Islands	5
United States of America	76,670
Uruguay	26
Venezuela	207
Total	**88,233**

Western Europe

Country	*Number of cases*
Austria	211
Belgium	368
Denmark	319
Finland	32

175

France	4,211
Germany, Federal Republic of	2,488
Greece	127
Iceland	6
Ireland	49
Italy	2,556
Luxembourg	12
Malta	12
Monaco	1
Netherlands	605
Norway	91
Portugal	173
San Marino	–
Spain	1,471
Sweden	223
Switzerland	502
United Kingdom	1,794
Total	15,251

Eastern Europe

Country	Number of cases
Albania	–
Bulgaria	3
Czechoslovakia	11
German Democratic Republic	6
Hungary	14
Poland	3
Romania	8
USSR	4
Yugoslavia	40
Total	89

Asia

Country	Number of cases
Afghanistan	–
Bahrain	–
Bangladesh	–
Bhutan	–
Brunei Darussalam	–
Burma	–
China	3
China (Province of Taiwan)	1
Cyprus	5
Democratic People's Republic of Korea	–
Democratic Yemen	–
Hong Kong	13
India	9
Indonesia	3
Iran	–
Iraq	–
Israel	65
Japan	90
Jordan	3
Kuwait	1
Lebanon	5
Malaysia	4
Maldives	–
Mongolia	–
Nepal	–
Oman	6
Pakistan	6
Philippines	17
Qatar	21
Republic of Korea	3
Singapore	4
Sri Lanka	1
Syrian Arab Republic	4
Thailand	8
Turkey	9
Viet Nam	–
Yemen	–
Total	**281**

Oceania

Country	Number of cases
Australia	1,024
Cook Islands	–
Fiji	–
French Polynesia	1
Kiribati	–
Mariana Islands	–
New Caledonia and Dependencies	–
New Zealand	89
Papua New Guinea	4
Samoa	–
Solomon Islands	–
Tonga	1
Tuvalu	–
Vanuatu	–
Total	1,119

*After revising their cases from 35 to 9, the Gambia has now reported 52 cases.
†The Malawian High Commissioner in London denies that Malawi has this number of cases.

Glossary

African swine fever	A viral infection of pigs
AIDS	Acquired immune deficiency syndrome.
AIDS related complex (ARC)	A condition of prolonged fever, severe weight loss, and persistent malaise and lethargy caused by infection with the AIDS virus.
Amoebiasis	Infection with a single celled parasite called *Entamoeba histolytica*.
Anergy	Absence of reaction of cell-mediated immunity, usually referring to a lack of reaction to substances injected into the skin.
Ankylostomiasis	Hookworm infestation.
Antibody	Serum protein produced by the body to fight infection.
Antigen	A substance which can stimulate the body to make an immune response, eg to produce antibodies.
Aplastic pancytopaenia	A condition where the body no longer produces white blood cells.
Appendicitis	Inflammation of the appendix.
Arthralgia	Pain affecting the joints.
Ascaridiasis	Infestation with the Ascaris worm.
Asymptomatic	Without symptoms

179

Atypical	Not typical
Auto-antibodies	An antibody that reacts with the patient's own tissues rather than a foreign substance eg bacteria.
Autopsy	Post-mortem
Biopsy	Examination of tissue removed from the living body.
B-lymphocyte	A type of lymphocyte that, when stimulated by an antigen, becomes a plasma cell and produces antibodies.
Bronchoalveolar lavage	Washing out of the lungs by passing fluid down the air passages.
Bronchopneumonia	Infectious inflammation of the lungs and bronchioles (small air passages).
Burkitt's lymphoma	An unusual type of malignant tumour of lymphoid tissue, relatively common in children in tropical Africa.
Cachexia	An extreme state of general ill-health with wasting.
Candida albicans	A yeast-like fungus.
Candidiasis	Infection with *Candida albicans.*
Cell-mediated immunity	An immune response to infection mediated by special types of white blood cells called T-lymphocytes.
Chemotherapy	Treatment of malignant disease with potent drugs.
Chorioretinitis	Inflammation of the choroid and retina, sensitive tissue at the back of the eye.
Cryptococcosis	A disease caused by *Cryptococcus neoformans,* frequently an opportunistic infection.
Cryptococcus neoformans	A yeast-like fungus.
Cutaneous	Of the skin.
Cytomegalovirus	A member of the herpes virus group.
Demography	The study of populations.
Dermatitis	Inflammation of the skin.

Dermatologist	A specialist in skin diseases.
Disseminated	Dispersed or spread throughout an organ, tissue or the whole body.
Ebola virus	A virus which causes a haemorrhagic fever.
ELISA	Enzyme Linked Immunosorbent Assay, a type of antibody test.
Encephalitis	Inflammation of the brain.
Endemic	Referring to a disease or infection caused by factors constantly present in the affected community.
Epidemiology	The study of the prevalence and spread of a disease in a population.
Factor VIII	A blood protein necessary for blood clotting, deficient in patients with haemophilia.
Filariasis	Infection with worms from the family Filarioidea.
Fulminant	Developing suddenly.
Haematogenous	Transported by the blood.
Haemophilia	A severe hereditary bleeding disease of males but transmitted by females.
Helminthic	Pertaining to worms.
Helper T-cells (T4 cells)	A type of T-lymphocyte that controls the responses of killer T-lymphocytes and B-lymphocytes.
Hepatitis A and B	Inflammation of the liver caused by virus types A and B.
Hepatosplenomegaly	Enlargement of the liver and spleen.
Herpes simplex	A virus, member of the Herpes virus group, that causes cold sores and other infections.
Herpes zoster	A virus, member of the Herpes virus group, that causes chicken pox and shingles.
Histopathology	Microscopic description or investigation of diseased tissues.

HIV	Human immunodeficiency virus, the virus responsible for AIDS.
HLA	Name for the major histocompatibility antigens in humans, an individual's genetically determined tissue type.
Holoendemic	A term used to describe areas where malaria infection is particularly intense.
Homophobia	Fear of or aversion to homosexuality.
HTLV-I	Human T-Lymphotropic Virus type I that causes a type of leukaemia.
HTLV-II	Human T-Lymphotropic Virus type II. This virus is not known to cause disease.
HTLV-III	Human T-Lymphotropic Virus type III. This is the original American name for the AIDS virus, now called HIV.
Hyperendemic	A term applied to a highly endemic area.
Hypothesis	A proposition made as a basis for reasoning, without assumption of its truth.
Idiopathic	Describing any pathological condition of unknown cause.
Immunity	The state of resistance of the body to disease, particularly infection.
Immune system	The body's defence system. It recognizes and neutralises or destroys 'foreign' invaders such as bacteria, viruses, fungi and parasites, and also destroys malignant cells.
Immunology	The study of immunity.
Immunodeficiency	A deficiency of the immune system that can be inherited, or can be caused by certain drugs, malignant disease, infections or other factors.

Immunofluorescence	A technique of labelling specially prepared antibodies with fluorescent dyes.
Immunosuppression	The suppressing, wholly or in part, of the body's immune responses.
Inguinal	Groin eg extra-inguinal lymphadenopathy, lymph nodes outside the groin region.
Interstitial pneumonia	An uncommon type of pneumonia
Kaposi's sarcoma	A malignant disease that usually affects the skin of the limbs but may also affect internal organs.
Lassa fever	A viral illness spread by rodents, first described in Nigeria.
LAV	Lymphadenopathy associated virus, the original French name for the AIDS virus, now called HIV.
Legionaire's disease	A type of pneumonia caused by a bacteria spread by air conditioning systems.
L. donovani	*Leishmania donovani,* the parasite that causes leishmaniasis.
Leishmaniasis	Diseases caused by a single celled parasite, *L. donovani*. Three disease entities occur, visceral leishmaniasis or kala-azar, mucocutaneous leishmaniasis, and cutaneous leishmaniasis.
Leucopaenia	A diminution in the number of white blood cells.
Leukaemia	Malignant disease of the white blood cells.
Leukemoid	Resembling leukaemia.
Lymph nodes	Small oval or bean-shaped bodies composed chiefly of lymphocytes.
Lymphadenopathy	Enlargement of lymph nodes that may be widespread (generalised) or localised.
Lymphocytes	A type of white blood cell that plays an important part in the immune response.

Lymphoma	A general term comprising tumours arising from some or all of the cells of lymphoid tissue. In undifferentiated lymphoma the type of cell giving rise to the tumour cannot be identified.
Lymphoreticular	Pertaining to lymphoid and reticular cells.
Maculopapular	Characterised by maculae (a circumscribed alteration in skin colour) and papules (small, raised skin lesions).
Malignant	Threatening life or tending to cause death. Used to describe tumours that spread throughout the body.
Marburg virus	Virus of unknown origin responsible for outbreaks of disease amongst laboratory workers in Marburg, Germany.
Meningitis	Inflammation of the membranes surrounding the brain and spinal cord.
Miliary	Of the size of a millet seed.
Miliary tuberculosis	Tuberculosis spread via the blood stream causing multiple small tuberculous granulomas.
Monocyte	A type of white blood cell.
Mucocutaneous	Relating to mucous membranes and the skin.
Mucosa	Mucous membrane; the moist membrane lining the mouth, nose, sinuses, gut, air passages and other structures.
Multifocal	Occurring in a number of different sites.
Mutation	A sudden change of the genetic material of the cell which affects its function.
Mycobacterium tuberculosis	Bacterium causing tuberculosis in man.
OKT4/OKT8 ratio (T4/T8 ratio)	The ratio between T-helper and T-suppressor lymphocytes,

	normally about 2.4:1.
Oesophageal	Relating to the oesophagus, or food pipe.
Onchocerciasis	Infestation with a type of filarial worm that causes severe damage to the skin and eyes.
Opportunistic infection	Infection by a commonly occurring microorganism which does not usually cause disease except when the immune system is seriously impaired.
Oral	Belonging to the mouth.
Parenteral	Introduced into the body by any route other than the digestive tract.
Parasitaemia	Parasites circulating in the blood stream.
Pathogen	Any living organism or other agent which is the cause of disease.
Pathogenesis	The production and development of diseased conditions.
Pathologist	A specialist in the study of the dead body.
Perianal condylomata	Wart-like lesions around the back passage.
Plasmodium falciparum	Malarial parasite responsible for the commonest type of malaria.
Pneumocystis carinii	A commonly occurring micro-organism of uncertain classification that normally only causes disease when immunity is impaired.
Pneumococcus	A bacteria that can cause pneumonia and other infections.
Pneumonia	Severe infection of the lung.
Polymorphous	Relating to or existing in a number of distinct forms.
Prodrome, adj prodromal	An early premonitory symptom which is not infrequently of a different nature from the symptoms of the true onset of the disease.

185

Protozoal	Pertaining to or caused by protozoa (single celled parasites).
Pruritic	Itchy.
Radiography	X-ray photography.
Radio-immunoassay	A type of antibody assay using radioactively labelled antigen.
Radio-immunoprecipitation	A variant of radio-immunoassay.
Retrovirus	The group of viruses that includes the AIDS virus (HIV), HTLV-I and II, and the Lenti viruses that cause degenerative brain disease in sheep and goats.
Salmonella	A group of bacteria causing typhoid fever, paratyphoid fever and food poisoning.
Schistosomiasis	Bilharziasis; A group of diseases caused by parasites, in whom an essential stage of the life cycle is passed through snails.
Septicaemia	A severe type of infection in which the blood stream is invaded by large numbers of bacteria.
Seroepidemiology	The study of the incidence of an infection in a defined population by testing for serum antibodies in a sample of the population.
Serology (adj serological)	The study of blood sera.
Seropositive (true and false)	Giving a positive reaction to serological tests. If the test is not specific, it may respond to more than one antibody and give a false positive result.
Serum (plural sera)	The yellowish fluid that remains after whole blood or plasma has been allowed to clot. It will contain all the antibodies in the blood sample.
Splenomegaly	Enlargement of the spleen.
Stomatitis	Inflammation of the mucous membrane of the mouth.
Suppressor T-cells	A type of T-lymphocyte that suppresses antibody production by activated B-lymphocytes

(plasma cells).

T-lymphocytes — Lymphocytes are a type of small white blood cell. There are two main types, T-lymphocytes which are responsible for cell mediated immunity, and B-lymphocytes that produce antibody. T-lymphocytes are particularly susceptible to infection with the AIDS virus.

Toxoplasma gondii — A single celled parasite causing a congenital or acquired infection that frequently affects the nervous system.

Toxoplasmosis (cerebral) — Toxoplasma infection in the brain, usually a reactivation of a previous, dormant infection.

Trypanosomiasis — The diseases caused by infection with a type of single celled parasite. The African form is commonly called sleeping sickness and is transmitted by the tsetse fly.

Tuberculin — An extract of the tubercule bacillus (the bacteria that causes tuberculosis).

Vector — An animal eg mosquito which carries other organisms, particularly parasites, from one host to another.

Western blot — A test for AIDS antibodies. It is more reliable than the ELISA test but still gives false positive results.

Selective Index

This edition of
AIDS, Africa and Racism
was finished in March 1989.

It was printed on a Miller TP 41,
on 80g/m^2 vol. 18 book wove.

The new material for this edition
was commissioned by Robert M. Young,
edited by Les Levidow
and produced by Martin Klopstock and Selina O'Grady
for Free Association Books.